W0019009

Health Disparities and the Applied Linguist

Maricel G. Santos, Rachel Showstack, Glenn Martínez, Drew Colcher, and Dalia Magaña

with an Afterword by Pilar Ortega

Routledge
Taylor & Francis Group
NEW YORK AND LONDON

First published 2023
by Routledge
605 Third Avenue, New York, NY 10158

and by Routledge
4 Park Square, Milton Park, Abingdon, Oxon, OX14 4RN

Routledge is an imprint of the Taylor & Francis Group, an informa business

© 2023 Taylor & Francis

The right of Maricel G. Santos, Rachel Showstack, Glenn Martínez, Drew Colcher, and Dalia Magaña to be identified as authors of this work has been asserted in accordance with sections 77 and 78 of the Copyright, Designs and Patents Act 1988.

All rights reserved. No part of this book may be reprinted or reproduced or utilised in any form or by any electronic, mechanical, or other means, now known or hereafter invented, including photocopying and recording, or in any information storage or retrieval system, without permission in writing from the publishers.

Trademark notice: Product or corporate names may be trademarks or registered trademarks, and are used only for identification and explanation without intent to infringe.

Library of Congress Cataloging-in-Publication Data
Names: Santos, Maricel Guiao, author. | Showstack, Rachel, author. | Martínez, Glenn A., 1971– author. | Colcher, Drew, author. | Magaña, Dalia, author. | Ortega Hernández, Mária del Pilar, writer of afterword.
Title: Health disparities and the applied linguist / Maricel G. Santos, Rachel Showstack, Glenn Martínez, Drew Colcher, Dalia Magaña ; with afterword by Pilar Ortega.
Description: New York, NY : Routledge, 2023. | Includes bibliographical references and index. |
Identifiers: LCCN 2022038443 (print) | LCCN 2022038444 (ebook) | ISBN 9780367484712 (hardback) | ISBN 9781032429540 (paperback) | ISBN 9781003041184 (ebook)
Subjects: LCSH: Communication in medicine—United States. | Health services accessibility—United States. | Medicine—Language | Discrimination in language—United States. | Discrimination in medical care—United States. | Applied linguistics—United States.
Classification: LCC R118 .S27 2023 (print) | LCC R118 (ebook) | DDC 610.1/4—dc23/eng/20221020
LC record available at https://lccn.loc.gov/2022038443
LC ebook record available at https://lccn.loc.gov/2022038444

ISBN: 9780367484712 (hbk)
ISBN: 9781032429540 (pbk)
ISBN: 9781003041184 (ebk)

DOI: 10.4324/9781003041184

Typeset in Times New Roman
by codeMantra

Contents

Figures

Tables

Acknowledgments

We would like to thank the Routledge editorial staff, Elysse Preposi and Harry Dixon, for their guidance and assistance. We also would like to thank Gayathri Tamilselvan for support with the manuscript editing and proofing. We are particularly grateful to Elysse, who first encouraged us to write this book and has continued to support our process, even after multiple pandemic-related setbacks. We appreciate the anonymous reviewers of our initial proposal whose input helped to shape the book's content.

We also extend our deep gratitude to Dr. Pilar Ortega, who generously accepted our invitation to read the book and write the Afterword. Dr. Ortega is a bilingual emergency physician, educator, author, and researcher at the University of Illinois College of Medicine with over 10 years of experience in health equity, diversity, and language justice throughout the continuum of medical education. She is also Founding President of the not-for-profit National Association of Medical Spanish. Dr. Ortega's feedback on an earlier draft of the book pushed our thinking about the syndemic view on health disparities, the implications for community engagement, and our positionalities.

Licensed material

Excerpts from *Spanish in Health Care: Policy, Practice, and Pedagogy in Latino Health* by Glenn Martínez, New York: Routledge, 2020. Reproduced with permission of The Licensor through PLSclear.

1 Language, health disparities, and applied linguistics[1]

By the end of this chapter, you will be able to answer these questions:

1. What do we mean when we say "language is a social determinant of health"?
2. How has the syndemic lens helped to deepen our understanding of how social and economic conditions shape the healthcare outcomes of linguistically diverse communities?
3. Why is our understanding of language critical to our ability to understand and dismantle healthcare disparities?

Introduction

"Language opens doors."

As a language teacher or a language learner, you are likely to have come across this well-worn aphorism. It highlights the fact that language has transformative potential. Language affects the way we live our lives: the languages and dialects that we speak shape who our friends are, what we read, the ease with which we travel abroad, the type of job we have, who we choose to be our partner, or how we raise our children. Language is a fundamental part of our lives.

How, then, does the language we speak affect our health and health care? To describe the relationship between language and health is no easy undertaking. A novice might approach the question wondering how a person's vocabulary and grammar could impinge on the presence of illness in that individual. However, such

DOI: 10.4324/9781003041184-1

an approach would miss much of the larger conceptualization of both language and health. The World Health Organization (WHO), as early as 1946, adopted a definition of health that encompasses much more than the absence of disease. According to the WHO, "health is a state of complete physical, mental, and social well-being and not merely the absence of disease or infirmity" (WHO, n.d., para. 1). By this definition, the question of the relationship between language and health requires attention to diseased states but also to the myriad factors affecting physical, mental, and social well-being. **Health equity** is "achieved when every person has the opportunity to 'attain his or her full health potential' and no one is 'disadvantaged from achieving this potential because of social position or other socially determined circumstances', including language" (Centers for Disease Control and Prevention, 2022, March 3).

In the same vein, a view of language as a specific set of lexical items (i.e., words or phrases) and grammatical rules used to communicate misses the mark of our current conceptualization of language. While Ferdinand de Saussure (2013) defined language as "a social product of our language faculty...[and] a body of necessary conventions adopted by society to enable members of society to use their language faculty" (p. 11), he was quick to distinguish this abstracted notion of "language" from "speech," which he characterized as "many-sided and heterogenous" and as belonging both to the individual and society. Saussure bracketed off speech from his consideration because he found that in speech, there was no unity to be discovered. This same division was held well into the twentieth century and became a foundational tenet of at least one variety of linguistic science. By bracketing off real-life use of language as speech and considering the underlying "system" of language as the only appropriate object of language science, linguists ignored the real consequences of language in social life. In this way, any attempt to understand the relationship between language and health care remained out of scope for language scientists.

This book is made possible because a whole field of language study, sociolinguistics, is dedicated principally to understanding how language is used in social contexts for social purposes. Dell Hymes (1997) referred to this approach as "socially constituted linguistics," in which all questions about language are to some extent embedded in social analysis. Hymes' pioneering ideas, in conjunction with those proposed by a long line of other scholars, have considerably expanded our notion of what language is and what it means to use and acquire it. From the tradition of sociolinguistic scholarship, a range of perspectives on language have emerged, including the study of language variation, language stylization, language attitudes and ideologies, language maintenance and shift – the list continues. What is clear from the legacy of sociolinguistics is that the relationship between language and health is a rich, complex, and multi-faceted area of linguistic inquiry.

Language is the vehicle through which patients and clinicians give and receive information. Without a shared communication system, access to care will be limited. At the same time, poorly designed access curtails the patient's ability to obtain information that is critical for understanding their condition, symptoms, treatment options, and possible risk factors. Limited access to information and care is perhaps the most obvious adverse effect of language barriers.

For policy-makers and health equity advocates, an obvious solution to language barriers is using trained, professional interpreter staff to bridge the information gap between patients and providers. The field of medical interpreting has grown substantially since the 1990s and today constitutes a vital service for patients with non-English language preference in the U.S. health delivery system (Ortega et al., 2022). To ensure the quality of interpreted medical encounters, the medical interpreting profession has developed standards of practice and ethical guidelines (Bancroft et al., 2016). The provision of professional interpretation services in the care of non-English-speaking patients has rapidly become the standard of care (U.S. Department of Health and Human Services Office of Minority Health, 2001, 2013; The Joint Commission, 2010). In addition to the professionalization of the interpreter role, investing in our bilingual healthcare workforce can result in more clinicians who are able to speak directly to patients in their preferred language. Recent efforts are moving toward a standardized process of training, validating, and using bilingual health professionals (Ortega, 2018; Tang et al., 2011).

Beyond improving communication between English-speaking providers and their non-English-speaking patients, there are other ways in which language plays a role in health and health care. As demonstrated by the seminal work of Shirley Brice Heath (1983), language can forge bonds of trust and connection between speakers, which are vital to any patient-provider relationship. It also signals relations of power and authority, because certain ways of speaking and using language hold value in specific contexts. Bourdieu (1991) described language as a form of **symbolic capital** that establishes and perpetuates social hierarchies (Bourdieu, 1991). Through language, people fashion their identities, adjusting their language to signal affiliation to different social groups (Rampton, 2018). These insights into the identity function of language suggest that language differences are never neutral but always charged with deep-seated, heart-felt meaning.

In her classic work, *Borderlands/La Frontera*, feminist scholar-activist Gloria Anzaldúa underscored this point. "So, if you really want to hurt me," she wrote, "talk badly about my language. Ethnic identity is twin skin to linguistic identity – I am my language. Until I can take pride in my language, I cannot take pride in myself" (Anzaldúa, 1999, p. 81). Language is deeply personal. In her poem "You know how to say *arroz con pollo* but not what you are," poet Melissa Lozada-Oliva explores what it means to claim Spanish as her own. She writes:

> If you ask if I am fluent in Spanish I will tell you … My Spanish is understanding that there are stories that will always be out of my reach, there are people who will never fit together the way that I want them to, there are some letters that will always stay silent, there are some words that will always escape me.
>
> (Lozada-Oliva, 2017)

For Lozada-Oliva, language is fundamental not only to her identity but also to her personhood. Her Spanish is who she is.

This identity function of language, embedded as it is in a whole array of social hierarchies, racial and ethnic prejudices, and socio-cultural expectations, also impinges on the relationship between language and health. If the communicative function of language limits *access* to health care, the identity function of language limits and strains *acceptance* in health care. It is not enough simply to have access to information. There is also a need to feel accepted, welcomed, and justly heard in the healthcare encounter. Lack of acceptance leads to mistrust between patients and providers and has the potential to override any gains realized through access. Lack of acceptance, moreover, shapes the dispositions of both the clinician and the patient. Perhaps a patient's lack of compliance or leaving the hospital against medical advice (Desai et al., 2016) is nothing more than a symptom of a lack of trust. Perhaps a clinician's over-utilization of costly tests and increased worries about medical malpractice lawsuits in treating linguistically minoritized patients stems from a lack of acceptance (Chen et al., 2011).

The use of interpreters, however, does little to mitigate the barriers of acceptance occasioned by communication gaps. Telephonic interpreter, Nataly Kelly, for example, describes how her mediation skills, even while effective in closing an access gap, were useless in bridging the gap of acceptance. She writes:

> I've witnessed – by phone – some behavior by providers that is offensive or rude. I've interpreted for patients who ask, "Why is the doctor speaking so slowly to me? Does he think I'm stupid?" I've also interpreted the words, "Please tell the nurse not to yell at me. I don't have a hearing problem – I just don't speak English." Recently I heard a physician say, in all seriousness, "Next time you come, you speak *inglés*, understand?" as if mastery of a new language would magically occur by the follow-up appointment.
>
> (Kelly, 2008, p. 1704)

As Kelly's observations illustrate, the interpreter alone does not bear the burden of removing barriers to language-appropriate care. Some have argued that training healthcare providers to work with an interpreter is needed (Diamond & Jacobs, 2010). Others have contended that successfully confronting these issues requires training in cultural competence (Watt et al., 2016). While both are promising interventions, it is important to realize that language acceptance is part of a much larger habitus in which health care is couched. **Habitus** is a concept developed by Bourdieu as part of a more complex theory of practice. He speaks of the habitus as "systems of durable, transposable dispositions" that are deployed in "regulated and regular" form without being "the product of the orchestrating action of a conductor" (Bourdieu, 1990, p. 53). Habitus thus refers to values, attitudes, ideologies, and actions that are adopted unconsciously as part of membership in a particular field. With respect to language, we might conceive of a series of dispositions about what is considered normative language in clinical spaces. Those dispositions are challenged when a doctor must dial a phone and connect to an interpreter to converse with a patient. The dissonance can result in the type of encounter chronicled by Kelly.

Seth Holmes (2013), in his ethnography of Oaxacan migrant farmworkers, argues that cultural competency training models often fail to adequately frame the problem of the larger habitus. He contends that most training programs focus on lists of stereotypical cultural traits and thus implicitly portray cultural difference as the problem. Building on the work of Jonathan Metzl, Holmes argues that medical educators should shift their focus to social analysis and structural competency rather than on cultural competency (p. 153). In other words, the primary driver of unequal care is not so much the culture that patients and providers bring with them to the encounter but rather the structures in which those cultures are embedded and activated. Critical reflection about the structures or habitus that give meaning to linguistic and cultural practices will no doubt improve practices in applied linguistics and health care.

Tervalon and Murray-García (1998) view cultural humility as an alternative to cultural competency that would address the larger habitus of health care. **Cultural humility** attempts to reframe competence as a disposition to approach other cultures with a pervasive desire to learn; it is listening attentively and not assuming a shared perspective. While **cultural competence** is often characterized as a set of skills and practices that an individual practitioner strives to master, cultural humility is rooted in relationship, a practice that builds connection to others that must be nurtured and reinforced.

Tervalon and Murray-García's (1998) work in healthcare settings provides an example of the differences between cultural competence and cultural humility. They describe the experience of a Spanish-dominant speaking Latina patient who is complaining of excruciating pain after a surgical procedure. The patient is seen by an English-dominant speaking doctor in the presence of a Latina nurse. The doctor is concerned about the patient's pain. The nurse, however, replies that Latinas generally exaggerate their pain and that she is probably fine with the current level of pain medication. In this case, the nurse is presenting herself as culturally competent but not culturally humble. Oblivious to the power imbalances in the encounter, the nurse fails to see how her stance as the "cultural expert" undermines the patient's legitimate request for additional pain medication. Finally, the institution takes no responsibility for its complicitness: the doctor simply agrees with the nurse without any further reflection, probing, or exploration.

Cultural humility is a necessary intervention to promote diversity, equity, and inclusion in health care, but adopting the concept should not displace the focus on cultural competence. Recent debates suggest that cultural competence and humility complement each other (Nguyen et al., 2021; Stubbe, 2020). While cultural humility is an approach for engaging across cultures, cultural competence is the product of ongoing reflection and learning. Given the complexities of cultures that are influenced by numerous social factors, cultural competence should be viewed as a process of on-going inquiry that unfolds across the life span, not a finite set of skills and knowledge (see Chapter 4). As noted earlier, trying to map the complexity of social factors that shape our healthcare experiences is an enormous task. No doubt this ongoing inquiry into our own capacity to provide culturally responsive health care will yield a richer, deeper, arguably more valuable understanding of the relationship between language, health, and power. We now invite the reader to enter this line of inquiry.

The social determinants of health

The empirical study of how language preference and use impact health disparities has evolved considerably over the past two decades. In the next two sections, we consider the evolution of this empirical research, identify gaps, and propose alternative theoretical insights that may provide new understandings of the place of language in health disparities. Rooted in social epidemiology, a subfield of epidemiology has emerged that seeks to uncover the influence of social circumstances on health, or what is widely termed **social determinants of health**, sometimes abbreviated SDOH. The U.S. Department of Health and Human Services (HHS) defines social determinants as "the conditions in the environments where people are born, live, learn, work, play, worship, and age that affect a wide range of health, functioning, and quality-of-life outcomes and risks" (n.d.).

The focus on social determinants forces us to rethink the popular assumption that good health results from people making good individual choices. The emphasis on individual choices – such as the choice to eat well, exercise, not smoke, get regular check-ups, or follow screening guidelines – may not seem controversial, but the problem is that it fails to account for the broader social, economic and physical environmental conditions that may influence the kinds of choices we are able to make. In other words, where we are born, live, work, go to school, or raise our families can make a significant difference in our health outcomes, quality of life, access to care, disease risk, and our sense of safety (Centers for Disease Control and Prevention, 2022).

For example, we understand that a diet high in saturated fat and salt can lead to a greater likelihood of a heart attack. From a social determinants view, we consider the reasons why some people are more likely than others to consume this type of high-risk diet. As Marmot (2005) has noted: "it is not an accident that people consume diets high in saturated fat and salt. It represents the nature of the food supply, culture, affordability, and availability, among other influences" (p. 3). These more distal influences, e.g., economic stability, education level, neighborhood, access to healthy food, are thus viewed as social determinants of health. A low-income neighborhood where people have easy access to fast food might have an unhealthier population than a neighborhood with access to affordable healthy food and safe recreation spaces.

The U.S. Department of Health and Human Services groups social determinants into five domains and offers examples of key issues:

1 economic stability – employment, food insecurity, and housing instability
2 education access and quality – early childhood education, enrollment in higher education, high school graduation, and language/literacy
3 healthcare access and quality – access to primary care and health literacy
4 neighborhood and built environment – access to foods that support healthy eating patterns, crime and violence, environmental conditions, and quality of housing
5 social and community context – civic participation, discrimination, incarceration, and social cohesion (based on U.S. Department of Health & Human Services, n.d.)

This is not intended to be a definitive list. In fact, in the past decade, there have been multiple attempts to refine and expand the taxonomy to account for the less visible factors and conditions that contribute to health disparities (Braveman & Gottleib, 2014). Referring to "language" as a social determinant of health can index efforts to improve low levels of English proficiency so that people can manage the communicative demands of our U.S. healthcare system, as well as the linguistic discrimination, isolation, and poor provision of care affecting linguistically minoritized groups. We agree with Islam (2019) that "perhaps it is wise to slightly modify the term and make it something like 'social determinants of health and related inequalities' so that it covers the *determinants of health* and the *determinants of inequalities in health*" (p. 2, italics in original).

Recently, researchers and advocates have argued that digital connectivity – broadly referring to our digital access and skills – is a **super social determinant of health** because connectivity appears to affect multiple other social determinants of health. How does one apply for housing assistance without online access? How digitally skilled is one expected to be to set up an appointment in a patient portal, fill a prescription, or seek a referral? To what extent are online tools making it easier or harder for linguistically minoritized groups to communicate with and build rapport with clinicians? During the COVID-19 pandemic, linguistically minoritized communities have experienced triple disadvantages due to poor linguistic access, low digital literacy, and poor telehealth infrastructures (Rodriguez et al., 2021).

In a call to action to members of the American Association for Applied Linguistics, Showstack et al. (2019) drew attention to health disparities suffered by linguistic groups, typically at the forefront of our teaching, research, and service commitments:

> Many of the populations we focus on in our research and practice as applied linguists—immigrants and refugees, indigenous peoples, racial and ethnic minority groups, among others—experience serious *health disparities*, or unfair differences in health outcomes, that can be traced to a history of social and linguistic segregation, discrimination against minority groups, and weak investment in the neighborhoods where they live.
>
> (n.p.)

Showstack et al. (2019) urge applied linguists to use their expertise to refine the conceptualization of "language as a social determinant," and ultimately, to increase public understanding of the many ways that language and health are linked. For example, studies have found that speaking a language other than English has been associated with a lower likelihood of receiving eligible treatment (Cheng et al., 2007) and preventative health services (Jacobs et al., 2005). Patients who report "limited English proficiency" have lower rates of vaccination (Haviland et al., 2011), are less likely to participate in health-promoting lifestyle activities (Hulme et al., 2003), are more likely to have extended hospital stays (John-Baptiste et al., 2004), and less likely to have full informed consent documentation in their medical records (Schenker et al., 2007).

Language concordance studies focus on the comparative effects of receiving healthcare treatment in one's preferred language

(**language concordance**) and receiving it in the dominant language, possibly with the assistance of a language mediator (**language discordance**). Patients with Type 2 diabetes, for example, who receive care in their first languages, are more similar to English-only speaking patients in terms of glycemic and LDL cholesterol control (Fernandez et al., 2011; Parker et al., 2017). Similarly, patients with cardiovascular disease who receive language-concordant care were more likely to adhere to their medication regimen than those who receive language-discordant care (Traylor et al., 2010). Patients with language-concordant clinicians are less likely to report confusion, frustration, or poor quality of care than those patients with language-discordant providers (González et al., 2010). Language concordance can support shared decision-making (Detz et al., 2014), patient questions (Jaramillo et al., 2016), and greater trust (Schenker et al., 2010).

Together these studies establish language as a social determinant or possibly a super social determinant of health. They show that language preference, use, and proficiency have a measurable impact on access to services and health outcomes. Further, they suggest that when language-concordant providers are present, health outcomes, quality of care, and intersubjective processes improve. Researchers, however, have begun to push the boundaries of these associations, raising questions about how language preference, use, and proficiency interact with other known social determinants of health and the influence of intersubjective processes beyond the language-concordant healthcare encounter.

The political determinants of health

Political action, policy making, and policy implementation also determine health outcomes. Daniel Dawes coined the phrase "**political determinants of health**" to refer to the determinants of the social determinants of health that reflect inequities of decision-making power (Dawes, 2020). Political actors, interest groups, and policies, Dawes argues, interact to create structures of exclusion and violence that generate health disparities. These structures of exclusion and violence are seen in political decisions against expanding Medicaid at the outset of implementing the Affordable Care Act, prohibitions on CDC research on gun violence, restrictions on organ transplant eligibility among immigrants, public charge clauses in immigration policy, and medical deportation.

We have seen in the previous section that interventions such as the use of interpreters and bilingual healthcare professionals can have a measurable impact on health outcomes. These interventions, however, are politically determined, a perspective we further explore in Chapter 2 where we examine the regulatory environment of language access to health care in the U.S. Political determinants also affect experiences with language acceptance that non-dominant English speakers face in the healthcare delivery system and in society at large. Anti-immigration rhetoric and its attendant draconian policies such as "show me your paper" laws, denying driver's licenses to undocumented individuals, and public charge immigration clauses generate a sense of fear and hiding that can exacerbate the effects of social determinants of health.

The syndemic viewpoint

Studies that seek to shed light on the interactions between language and other social and political determinants are beginning to uncover previously less visible connections. For example, researchers are beginning to look at mediating factors, such as racial identification and place of origin, that might affect the interaction between language and health (Abraído-Lanza, 2015; Cuevas et al., 2016). As Abraído-Lanza (2015) points out:

> Latino groups differ in sociopolitical histories and reasons for migrating to the United States. Moreover, the context of reception in the United States differs for the various groups and at different points as a result of economic conditions, labor shortages, and the political climate.
>
> (p. 567)

These differential contexts can shape the ways that language interacts with health. Economic conditions, labor shortages, and the political climate can significantly reduce the frequency of contact between Spanish-dominant speakers and health and social service agencies. For instance, a low-income Spanish speaker may not be able to afford to take time off from work to obtain preventative care. An undocumented worker may avoid health care due to lack of health insurance or fear of sharing personal information and deportation. Patient may not seek care if they fear discrimination for not speaking English (Cheng et al., 2018; Steinberg et al., 2016). These studies suggest that social determinants, including language, may be relative to the contexts in which they emerge and may depend on previous experiences. As communication scholar Elaine Hsieh (2018) has pointed out: "language discordance is situated in the complex tension of political power and linguistic legitimacy" (p. 3).

Researchers are also shifting focus to issues of intersubjectivity, prompting us to reflect on the links between language and health through the dimensions of the self, the other, and the world. Zlatev et al. (2008, cited in Thornbury, 2015, March 22) define **intersubjectivity** as "the sharing of experiential content (e.g., feelings, perceptions, thoughts, and linguistic meanings) among a plurality of subjects," claiming that "intersubjectivity is at the heart of what makes us human" (n.p.). Walqui (2006) recognizes intersubjectivity as an essential condition for meaningful interaction, focusing on the need for "mutual engagement and rapport" and "encouragement and non-threatening participation in a shared community of practice" (p. 165). Intersubjective processes can shape health outcomes and healthcare access. For example, a study of the beliefs and experiences of 20 Latina women in Utah, as they transitioned to a new society and healthcare system, found that the women expressed feelings of aloneness in seeking care. They recalled experiences with illness in their home countries as embedded in social worlds: the women's connections to various social networks, spanning intimate to official, supported access to care. But in the U.S., the loss of social support affected their ability to access care, as described by one woman in the study: "I feel that I could not defend myself in this country" (Sanchez-Birkhead et al., 2011, p. 1170). The researchers further noted that "limited time with and limited access to health providers… seemed to interfere with building the type of relationship with providers that women felt was needed" (p. 1172). In another study of language barriers among Latina mothers in Detroit and Baltimore, participants described navigating language barriers as a "battle," preferring care from bilingual providers and experiencing a negative bias toward interpreters; they reported trying to get by with limited English skills, fears of being a burden, stigma, and discrimination (Steinberg et al., 2016). These studies reveal the absence of shared "experiential content" between the self and others, and the additional stressors brought on by feelings of isolation and aloneness, struggles to access care, loss of social support, and othering. The ability of patients and clinicians to orient to one another, through language, gaze, attention, physical orientation, etc., is arguably a foundational condition of intersubjectivity, a phenomenon urgently needing more study and critical praxis in applied linguistics.

Studies on the interactions of language and other social determinants suggest that the effects of language preference, use, and proficiency are situated and contextual. Studies on the wider intersubjective processes affecting Spanish speakers, for example, indicate that language barriers interact with emotionally debilitating experiences both within the healthcare setting and beyond (Martínez, 2010, 2013, 2020). These approaches have in common their insistence on viewing language as couched in a larger set of processes that impact health outcomes and healthcare access. The social determinant model, however, has difficulty capturing how language is embedded in people's lived experience and how this experience also intersects with language with other social determinants, wider intersubjective processes, and, many times, co-occurring physical and mental health conditions (i.e., **co-morbidities**). The uni-directional nature of the social determinants model and its bias toward causation as opposed to interaction limits our ability to fully capture the multi-layered and complex relationship between, for example, being a speaker of Spanish and broadly termed "Latino health outcomes." The social determinant model does not fully capture the co-morbidities (e.g., diabetes and depression) that may occur among groups of Latino immigrants, which in turn are tied to issues of equity and social justice.

Syndemic theory is an alternative way to conceptualize the relationship between language and health in linguistically minoritized communities. Willen et al. (2017) emphasize the need for a new "idiom of social justice mobilization: a concrete strategy for melding scholarly insight and ethical values with the goal of promoting social justice in the health domain" (p. 965). Different disciplines contribute their own idioms to this justice work, e.g., international law focuses on health as a human right, but Willen et al. argue that "a rights based approach grounded in a syndemic sensibility offers an optimal framework" (p. 996) for bringing together disciplines and stakeholders across public and private sectors.

Rooted in medical anthropology, syndemic theory arose out of concerns around medical co-morbidities and the social factors that interacted with co-morbid conditions. Medical anthropologist Merrill Singer coined the term syndemic as a blend of the words synergy and epidemic to express the dominant focus of the approach on synergies in disease states. The concept emerged from Singer's work among HIV-AIDS patients in Connecticut. He found that most HIV-AIDS interventions that he encountered were designed primarily with middle-class, white, homosexual men in mind. These interventions were of little use in his work, where he encountered HIV-AIDS patients who not only did not match the demographic bias but also who were experiencing other conditions together with HIV-AIDS, namely substance abuse and violence. He thus set out to explore the experience of living with AIDS in conjunction with substance abuse and violence and characterized his work as focusing on the SAVA (Substance Abuse, Violence, AIDS) syndemic. He defines the term syndemic as "the concentration and deleterious interaction of two or more diseases or other health conditions in a population, especially as a consequence of social inequity and the unjust exercise of power" (Singer, 2009, p. xv).

Willen et al. (2017) further explain that social inequities in health care arise from

> the *negative feedback loop* among comorbidities and upstream factors that often are overlooked in routine clinical interactions—factors that include the social, economic, political, and structural determinants of health ... Any meaningful effort to tackle the 'deleterious clustering and interaction of diseases' faced by migrants, refugees, or other populations at risk must begin by mapping out the upstream determinants that interact to put certain individuals and groups in positions of syndemic vulnerability.
>
> (p. 965, emphasis added)

In this way, a **syndemic sensibility** moves us away from a focus on causation and invites us to focus instead on synergistic interactions.

The application of a syndemic sensibility can considerably advance our understanding of the relationship between language and health disparities. It invites us to contextualize language preference, use, and proficiency in ways that previous studies have overlooked. Further, it invites us to adopt a more granular perspective on language-concordant encounters. A syndemic sensibility in the study of language and health disparities, moreover, can open up new lines of research. For instance, how do life-course events and experiences shape and contribute to syndemic production? What role do prior childhood or recent immigrant experiences of linguistic othering play in the burden of disease within linguistically minoritized communities? Questions like these open up new lines of research and reflexive practice into the bi/multilingual experience in health care that currently is less visible or neglected.

Recap: Understanding different views on health disparities

We have seen that the relationship between language and health disparities has been approached from a variety of perspectives (see Figure 1.1). The social determinants of health model consider health disparities as the result of social determinants, including educational attainment, socioeconomic status, place of residence, etc. In this model, language can be seen as a super-determinant in as much as language proficiency is closely correlated with other social factors. The political determinants of health model, on the other hand, seek to account for health disparities and their corresponding social determinants from the perspective of political action and policy-making. Nothing inherently links place of residence, for example, to poorer health outcomes. Rather, the policies that shape the place of residence account for health disparities. For example, environmental policies that allow manufacturing plants to release dangerous levels of toxins into the environment make a place of residence less healthy. Economic policies that incentivize investments in convenience stores rather than grocery stores can also make a place of residence less healthy. Public safety policies that generate adversarial relationships between police and the community contribute to poor health outcomes in those neighborhoods. Policies, then, are what make a place of residence less healthy, and policies are formulated by political actors and interests. A syndemic approach, finally, suggests that the social and political determinants of health are not simply precursors to health disparities but instead shape a unique experience of poor health. If the social and political determinant models are an outside-in view of health disparities, the syndemic model is an inside-out view. Social and political determinants models seek to uncover the external factors that lead to health disparities. The syndemic model, on the other hand, seeks to display the insider's experience of disparity. From a syndemic perspective, it is not simply that place of residence causes untenable asthma exacerbations; rather it is that untenable asthma exacerbations are stacked onto an array of other conditions, including an unhealthy environment, low-wage employment, or limited educational opportunities: this stacking effect fundamentally shapes the experience of illness and well-being.

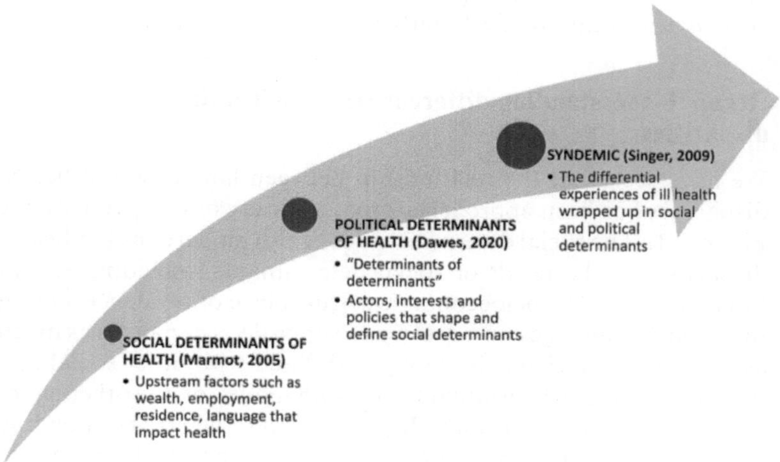

Figure 1.1 Different views on health disparities.

About this book

We began this book with an aphorism "language opens doors" to call attention to the transformative potential of language, but also, for many linguistically minoritized communities in the U.S., how the power afforded to English and not to other languages continues to contribute to suffering and health inequities. So much of this book rests on the hope that if applied linguists continue to engage in constructive interrogation of the link between language, power, and health, we will, indeed, be able to open doors: new thinking about the perceived and real power of English in our healthcare systems, new pathways for critical reflection on our **monolingual** (English only) **bias** in our healthcare practices and policies, new opportunities for the members of linguistically minoritized communities to speak for themselves and shape the solutions that are meant to ameliorate health disparities, and new routes of interchange between applied linguists and public health partners.

This book is inspired by our interdisciplinary work in a variety of contexts – Spanish heritage and second language education (Rachel Showstack, Glenn Martínez), clinical environments (Dalia Magaña, Glenn), Hispanic linguistics (Drew Colcher, Rachel, Dalia, Glenn), and adult English language/literacy education (Maricel Santos) – in collaboration with partners in public health and medicine. We are grateful to include, in the book's afterword, the perspective of a trained medical practitioner (Pilar Ortega) who champions health equity and language justice in medical education.

We are resolute that applied linguistics can and should help to reduce health disparities by working to elevate conversations about language, language use, and language users in health care. The book reflects the multiple hats we play in our fields of expertise – as faculty, scholars, teachers, activists, and community partners. At times, our writing takes on a scholarly tone as we synthesize health disparities research; other times, our writing conveys a strong tone of persuasion, an urgent call to action. Both approaches are intentional so that the reader is prompted to examine an essential question: to what extent can you use your expertise and tools to address the persistent health disparities in today's society?

Our primary goal is to provide the applied linguistics field with an introduction to health disparities and an overview of the different healthcare issues where applied linguists can make important contributions. Integrating theory and practice, the book examines how insights and tools in applied linguistics have been applied to research and interventions in multiple contexts: clinical interactions, language classrooms, and professional training programs, with references to influential research. Our intended readership is broad: students in language and linguistics programs, preprofessionals, as well as educators and administrators already working in language education practice and policy. In pursuit of cross-disciplinary dialogue, we also hope the book is read by public health, health education, or medical providers who seek to make language justice part of their professional practice.

This book highlights various areas of health disparities work that also reflect our experiences working with healthcare professionals and community partners. Chapter 1 has discussed different views on the interconnectedness of language, power, and health, and the research on U.S. health disparities, affecting linguistically minoritized communities. In Chapter 2, we provide a historical landscape for understanding U.S. health disparities and discuss key legislative policies addressing language access (e.g., Title VI of the Civil Rights Act of 1964, the Plain Writing Act of 2010), movements with direct implications for linguistic diversity, and recent shifts in linguistic ideology in health care. In Chapters 3–5, we explore three domains where applied linguists can help to advance health equity: healthcare professional training and education; clinical environments, and language classrooms. Chapter 6 reflects on our readiness to engage as community partners in health disparities work and offers recommendations for strengthening our capacity. In the book's Afterword, Pilar Ortega, a bilingual emergency physician, invites the reader to see language justice with new eyes, literally and symbolically, and then to take up action. Throughout the book, key concepts are highlighted in bold, to provide the reader with a starter glossary for talking about language and health equity. Each chapter ends with some questions for reflection and extension to fuel readers' imaginations about future career directions, questions for community-engaged research, and coalition-building.

Writing this book has professional and personal significance. Across our lifetimes, we have interacted with the healthcare system for a variety of reasons, including care for a teenage daughter with Type 1 Diabetes, long-distance care for elderly parents, interpreting for immigrant parents, care for a mother with breast cancer whose health beliefs and spiritual approach clash with the U.S. medical system, gender-affirming health care for a non-gender-conforming bilingual child, support for a family member who lives with a severe mental illness and chronic pain. Our universities, based in California, Kansas, and Texas, have ties to neighborhood communities with deep health disparities, made more acute during COVID-19. During the pandemic, we have been able to keep our jobs and access health care through employer-supported health insurance, but many in the communities we serve have not. In the two-year span, it took to hatch and write this book, the U.S. has lost over one million people to the pandemic – a level of staggering loss that defies comprehension, particularly because many of those deaths were preventable. We hope that the call to action echoed throughout this book honors all those we have lost during this global crisis and promises that, going forward, we will do better to dismantle inequities affecting linguistically diverse communities. We also hope this book signals our deep gratitude to our community partners, learners, educators, interpreters and translators, public health researchers, and clinicians who have continued to collaborate with us, even when the pandemic shutdown complicated our ability to continue the work.

Questions and activities

1 To what extent has the COVID-19 pandemic changed your thinking about the idea that good health results from people making good choices?

2 Think about a linguistically diverse locale you know and care a lot about, for example, the neighborhood where you grew up, or the city where you work or study. What are the social and economic conditions that seem to most affect people's ability to make healthy choices in that locale – such as housing, income levels, employment trends, transportation systems, digital connectivity, the way land is used or developed, or the quality of local schools? What signs do you see that these conditions affect the health outcomes of communities from different linguistic backgrounds?
3 Use the Internet or corpus (e.g., The Coronavirus Corpus) to find media coverage on healthcare experiences of a linguistic community you want to learn more about. Whose stories about health and well-being have been told about/in this community in the past year? What social determinants are highlighted, including any systemic barriers to language-appropriate care? Whose stories would you like to see given more coverage? Who in the community would you like to talk to? Who could you consult to learn more?

Note

1 This chapter includes modified excerpts from Martínez (2020) *Spanish in Health Care: Policy, Practice and Pedagogy in Latino Health*, with permission of The Licensor through PLSclear.

2 Health care and language in U.S. law

By the end of this chapter, you will be able to answer the following questions:

1. What legal documents ensure a patient's linguistic civil rights?
2. How are language-related regulations implemented and enforced? How are they not?
3. How can applied linguists work toward ensuring meaningful healthcare access?

Introduction

In 2017, two of this volume's authors attended a linguistics conference to present research on linguistic ideologies among Spanish speakers in Kansas. Part of their presentation described a lack of language services for Spanish speakers as a form of institutional discrimination. This included a paucity of interpreters in the local hospital and medical clinics relative to the area's more than 50% Latino population. A fellow attendee raised her hand and informed the presenters that, according to Title VI of the 1964 Civil Rights Act, all medical facilities that receive federal funding are required to accommodate the language needs of their patients. The hospital being discussed was theoretically violating federal law. Nearly the same incident occurred during a presentation at Wichita State University later that year: an informed attendee announced that these services are federally mandated. As with the previous attendee, this person expressed sadness and dismay at the fact that many healthcare providers are either unable or unwilling to offer the services required of them by U.S. law.

DOI: 10.4324/9781003041184-2

In the U.S., many healthcare providers do not fully consider the patient's perspective when providing services to diverse populations: that is, they do not prioritize **patient-centered care** (Gerteis et al., 2002). Patient-centered care is increasingly recognized as the most equitable and effective form of health care; it emphasizes an understanding of the patient's cultural and linguistic background – in addition to immediate medical needs – as crucial to health in a pluralistic society. To be successful, it therefore requires the empowerment of patients through language services and acceptance (Showstack, 2019a,b). This approach to medicine encourages practitioners to develop and inform the patient's active participation in the healthcare process, ultimately improving outcomes by working against physician paternalism (Cherny, 2012; Dunlap et al., 2015). Unfortunately, as the anecdotes above illustrate, not all medical workers adopt this approach.

The struggle for linguistic equity and equal services in U.S. health care is intimately tied to the history of political events and legislative decisions that establish language-related civil rights. These events and decisions simultaneously establish the legal responsibility of healthcare providers to offer "meaningful access" to services in a "culturally and linguistically appropriate manner" (U.S. Department of Health and Human Services Office of Minority Health, 2013). However, while providers are expected to accommodate the patient's language and cultural perspective, the legal definition of "meaningful access" is embedded in a web of political and ideological interpretations. Since individual institutions (like hospitals) are often allowed to define meaningful access for themselves, implementation is not universal, and longstanding barriers to healthcare access still exist for individuals with varying levels of fluency in American English (Chang & Fortier, 1998; Schiaffino et al., 2016).

"Limited English Proficient"

Among healthcare providers in the U.S., and in the related legal and scholarly literature, the term Limited English Proficient (LEP) describes patients who may face barriers accessing a federally funded service using only English. LEP was first used during the Supreme Court case *Lau v. Nichols, 1974* (Lindsay, 2005). It has since become the official designation for those who require language accommodations – such as an interpreter – from an agency that receives federal funding. This includes virtually all healthcare providers (The Joint Commission, 2010, p. 65), and there is a lengthy legal precedent requiring these institutions to accommodate the languages their patients speak.

The definition of LEP has been elaborated mainly by different departments of the federal government, like the Department of Justice (DOJ) and the Department of Health and Human Services (HHS). In 2000, HHS's Office for Civil Rights defined LEP as applying to those who "cannot speak, read, write or understand the English language at a level that permits them to interact effectively with healthcare providers and social service agencies" (U.S. Department of Health and Human Services Office for Civil Rights, 2000, p. 52763). The term actually describes a heterogeneous population representing many of the world's languages and ethnicities, as well as a range of English proficiencies far exceeding the false dichotomy of "proficient or not." Showstack et al. (2019) conclude that LEP simplifies linguistic reality and fails to adequately incorporate the patient's perspective.

However, in spite of its inherent inaccuracies and ethnocentric biases, the term LEP has been of some (not unproblematic) practical use to healthcare providers. In labeling patients LEP, organizations quantify the proportion of those they serve who are protected by Title VI of the Civil Rights Act. Simultaneously, they establish their responsibility to provide **meaningful access** to those groups. The Department of Justice defines providing meaningful access as

> …forbidding funding recipients… from "utiliz[ing] criteria or methods of administration which have the effect of subjecting individuals to discrimination because of their race, color, or national origin, or have the effect of defeating or substantially impairing accomplishment of the objectives of the program…"
>
> (2002)

This seemingly establishes federal legal protection against disparate levels of care based on racially and ethnically discriminatory practices. However, as discussed below, it fails to cite language as a specifically protected category, and operates on the assumption – backed by legal precedence – that nationality is a proxy for language. Along with many other factors, this lack of explicit language protection has contributed to a syndemic relationship (Diamond et al., 2019; Martínez, 2020) involving "Limited English Proficiency" and disparate outcomes in cases of breast cancer (Jacobs et al., 2005; Kamimura et al., 2016), diabetes (Chao et al., 2015; Fernandez et al., 2011), mental health care (Sentell et al., 2007; Snowden & McClellan, 2013), and more. That is, being categorized as LEP co-occurs with significant increases in risk for these conditions, placing millions of patients at an immediate disadvantage within the healthcare system despite ostensible legal protections.

To understand patients' language rights and why they are unevenly protected or enforced, it will be necessary to outline how American legal history positions those with LEP within the healthcare system.

Historical overview

The 1964 Civil Rights Act

Despite the ratification of the Reconstruction Amendments in the late nineteenth century – and the many meaningful victories won in the interim by feminist, labor, and anti-racist movements – the first significant civil rights legislation in the U.S. was the 1964 Civil Rights Act (Bourne, 2014; Rosenbaum & Schmucker, 2017). Far-reaching in scope, the Act addressed the fact that most minoritized communities in 1960s America were still actively and openly denied equal access to education, health care, voting services, and other basic civil rights. It prohibits discrimination on the basis of "race, color, religion, sex, or national origin" in any context involving employment, the federal government, and any agencies receiving government funding. In doing so, the Civil Rights Act more firmly establishes the unconstitutionality of official segregation and discrimination based on a variety of sociodemographic factors, a process which arguably began with the 1954 Supreme Court case *Brown v. Board of Education of Topeka* (Reardon & Owens, 2014) and continues today.

Particularly significant in discussions of language access is **Title VI** of the Civil Rights Act: "Non-discrimination in Federally Assisted Programs." This title establishes that any recipient of federal funds (via grants, contracts, or loans) must abide by the guidelines of the Act, or risk losing that funding. Since most healthcare providers receive federal funds in some way (principally through Medicare and Medicaid reimbursements), they fall under the jurisdiction of Title VI (Metzger, 1993). However, the Civil Rights Act does *not* afford protections for patients based on language, covering only "race, color, religion, sex, and nationality." Specific **linguistic civil rights** protections would arise through subsequent court rulings and legal interpretations of Title VI.

Lau v. Nichols

The first Supreme Court case to apply Title VI protections to language – *Lau v. Nichols, 1974* – addressed discrimination within a large school district in San Francisco. A group of over 2,000 Chinese students brought a suit against the district, arguing that providing English-only education constituted a form of **linguistic discrimination**, and a violation of Title VI of the Civil Rights Act (Moran, 2005). Despite the fact that many Spanish-speaking students suffered similar discrimination in the same school district, Edward Steinman – the Lau family's lawyer – felt that the public would be more sympathetic to "*Lau*, not *Lopez*," revealing some of the racial dynamics implicit in language rights debates in the U.S. (Moran, 2009). However, he also emphasized that some level of bilingual education existed for Spanish speakers, which was not the case for the Chinese community. Steinman and the students he represented proved that the lack of linguistically appropriate educational services had a "disparate impact" on their educational outcomes, and was therefore illegally discriminatory (Tran & Bhattarai, 2014). Prohibitions against discrimination by **disparate impact** – meaning programs or institutions that nullify Title VI protections in practice, despite ostensible compliance – were first laid out by the now-defunct Department of Health, Education, and Welfare (*ibid*), and significantly informed *Lau v. Nichols*.

The landmark case ultimately became a test of the Department of Education's Office for Civil Rights' attempts to broaden the scope of civil rights protections by including language as a protected category (Margulies, 1981). In establishing "national origin" as a legal and constitutional proxy for language, the *Lau v. Nichols* decision laid the groundwork for official federal protections for speakers of languages other than English throughout all 15 executive departments of the President's Cabinet. This decision does not specifically address health care, but rather protects the rights of people seeking assistance from any recipient of federal funding, including many healthcare-providing institutions. Like the Civil Rights Act, it represents only a partial (and in this case, mostly indirect) expansion of language access in health care.

Executive Order 13166

Executive Order 13166 was issued in 2000 under the Bill Clinton Presidential Administration (U.S. Department of Justice, 2000), and is arguably the next significant federal development of linguistic civil rights after *Lau v. Nichols*. It requires all federally funded institutions to examine their language accommodations, establish areas of weakness, and report steps for remedying barriers to access. It also establishes the Interagency Working Group on Limited English Proficiency (https://lep.gov), a DOJ repository for information on language rights within health care, and language-related healthcare complaints. In 2003, President George Bush upheld EO 13166 and issued additional guidelines (DeCola, 2011). In 2011, Attorney General Eric Holder released a memorandum to the heads of all federal agencies reaffirming the mandates of the executive order (Holder, 2011). As of the writing of this volume, it remains in force.

However, there has been relatively little legislation upholding 13166 and requiring the provision of meaningful healthcare access. This is because, as an Executive Order rather than a law, it lacks significant legal force (Tran & Bhattarai, 2014). It also fails to clearly define "meaningful" access, and subsequently, various departments published guidelines and handbooks to establish the term's parameters. HHS published "Policy guidance on the prohibition against national origin discrimination as it affects persons with Limited English Proficiency" in the *Federal Register* (2000). Here, the Department outlines "The four keys to Title VI compliance in the LEP context," describing how recipients of federal funds can ensure meaningful access and therefore be compliant with the Civil Rights Act (pp. 52766–52769). The document emphasizes:

1 *Assessment* of the language needs of the population to be served
2 *Development of comprehensive written policy* on language access
3 *Training of staff* to ensure understanding of how to carry out policies
4 *Vigilant monitoring* to ensure that LEP persons can meaningfully access the program

In 2002, the DOJ developed a related "4-factor analysis" for federal aid recipients (U.S. Department of Justice, 2002) to help determine what language accommodations they must offer their clients in pursuing meaningful access. The four factors are:

1 Demographics (the number of LEP patients likely to be seen)
2 Frequency (the regularity with which those patients are likely to be seen)

3. Nature of the program (i.e., its importance to LEP communities based on demographic health profiles and statistics)
4. Availability of resources and costs (i.e., whether the provision of language services will create an "excessive financial burden")

In theory, healthcare-providing programs and institutions must individually establish what "meaningful" and "appropriate" access is in terms of these loosely defined criteria. In turn, the criteria have been widely adopted by healthcare providers, but carry little regulatory weight. Some (e.g., DeCola, 2011; Tran & Bhattarai, 2014) argue that the framework of legal guidelines based on EO 13166 and its related developments constitute a robust grounding for stronger enforcement. Others (Keers-Sanchez, 2003) argue that mandatory language services constitute an undue burden on physicians and care providers. As this debate evolves, interpretable guidelines – rather than mandatory requirements – are the norm.

CLAS standards

In 2001, as part of the push to clarify EO 13166's mandates regarding "meaningful access," the U.S. Department of Health and Human Services (2001) released a set of standards for "Culturally and Linguistically Appropriate Services" within health care (accessible at https://thinkculturalhealth.hhs.gov/clas). The Department's Office of Minority Health (OMH) later expanded on these standards, publishing the updated "blueprint for sustaining CLAS policy and practice" (U.S. Department of Health and Human Services Office of Minority Health, 2013). This 192-page document identifies language discordance as a primary cause of health disparities between different ethnic and socioeconomic groups. To remedy this discordance, OMH outlines 15 standards for providing culturally and linguistically appropriate services, thus showing agencies and institutions how to comply with Title VI. The principal standard is:

> [To p]rovide effective, equitable, understandable, and respectful quality care and services that are responsive to diverse cultural health beliefs and practices, preferred languages, health literacy, and other communication needs.
>
> (p. 31)

The other standards outline how to achieve this in the areas of "Governance, Leadership, and Workforce (Standards 2–4);"

"Communication and Language Assistance (Standards 5–8);" and "Engagement, Continuous Improvement, and Accountability (Standards 9–15)." Standards 5 through 8 regard language specifically; they emphasize that service providers must work toward being able to

- Offer language assistance to individuals who have LEP, at no cost to them.
- Inform all individuals of the availability of language assistance services clearly and in their preferred language, verbally and in writing.
- Ensure the competence of individuals providing language assistance, recognizing that the use of untrained individuals and/or minors as interpreters should be avoided.
- Provide easy-to-understand materials and signage in the languages commonly used by the populations in the service area.

In essence, CLAS standards elaborate on the guidelines associated with EO 13166. As such, they represent a significant improvement, outlining in detail how healthcare institutions should accommodate patients who have been designated LEP. These standards have been reaffirmed by various federal agencies, and adopted by most healthcare and educational institutions, and social service agencies, but still do not establish clear routes of enforcement. Many researchers argue that such a lack of explicit legislation related to language rights contributes to health disparities for LEP patients (Chen et al., 2007; Youdelman, 2008). For a more thorough analysis of the effectiveness of CLAS standards and related guidelines/documents, see Martínez (2013, 2020).

The Affordable Care Act

In 2010, Congress under President Barack Obama enacted the Patient Protection and Affordable Care Act, referred to widely as The Affordable Care Act (ACA). ACA represents a far-reaching and extremely complex reworking of the U.S. healthcare system, and as such, is too intricate to describe in detail here. It created a public health insurance marketplace, subsidized by federal funding to increase access to insurance for low-income populations (Oberlander, 2010). The controversial final version stipulated a penalty to be paid by individuals above certain income levels who did not have either publicly or privately provided health insurance. Over time, participation in the public healthcare marketplace has been weakened by legislative and corporate developments, as well as the rising costs of marketplace policies, and the future of ACA is currently in question (Willison & Singer, 2017).

However, ACA is pertinent to language rights in health care because Section 1557 – the Act's non-discrimination provision – includes a subsection on "Ensuring meaningful access for individuals with Limited English Proficiency." This subsection provides a clear outline for the LEP patients' rights and the responsibilities of the providers serving them (Hunt, 2016). It is perhaps the first explicit legal interpretation by the federal government of Title VI of the 1964 Civil Rights Act regarding linguistic discrimination. It clarifies that

> the prohibition on national origin discrimination requires covered entities to take reasonable steps to provide meaningful access to each individual with limited English proficiency who is eligible to be served or likely to be encountered within the entities' health programs and activities.
>
> (U.S. Department of Health and Human Services, 2020a)

More so than any previous pieces of legislation, this document clarifies several key concepts within linguistic civil rights and healthcare access; for example, Section 1557 defines:

- *LEP*: a person with LEP is an individual whose primary language for communication is not English and who has a limited ability to read, write, speak, or understand English
- *Reasonable steps* (i.e., *meaningful access*): language assistance services, such as oral language assistance or written translation

Section 1557 also provides clearer language than many previous documents regarding the precise responsibilities of those entities affected by Title VI and subsequent legal decisions ("covered entities"), who are required to:

- Post a notice of individuals' rights, among other information
- Post taglines in the top 15 languages spoken by LEP individuals in that state, indicating the availability of language assistance

Covered entities are also prohibited from "using low-quality video remote interpreting services or relying on unqualified staff [and/or] translators[1] when providing language assistance services," and are encouraged to "develop and implement a **language access plan** to ensure they are prepared to take reasonable steps to provide meaningful access to each individual that may require assistance" (U.S. Department of Health and Human Services, 2020b). However, as in the case of EO 13166, these standards are

> flexible and context-specific, taking into account factors such as the nature and importance of the health program and the communication at issue, as well as other considerations, including whether an entity has developed and implemented an effective language access plan.
>
> (ibid)

The dismantling of ACA

Section 1557 of ACA provides a poignant example of the tenuousness of linguistic civil rights protections. The final version of this section was ruled on by The Department of Health and Human Services' Office of Civil Rights in 2016, in the last year of the Barack Obama Administration. Almost immediately, groups like The Franciscan Alliance (now Franciscan Health, a Catholic health system operating 14 hospitals in Indiana and Illinois), along with eight state governments, sued HHS, arguing that the non-discrimination stipulations of Section 1557 required hospitals to perform federally subsidized gender affirmation surgeries and abortion procedures (Keith, 2020a). In June 2020, HHS under the Donald Trump Administration issued a new final rule (essentially an official federal re-interpretation) of the protections related to gender, sex, and language that are secured by this portion of ACA (U.S. Department of Health and Human Services, 2020b). Although still uncertain, this development has the potential to place the linguistic regulations defined by Section 1557 in question.

In early 2020, the Supreme Court ruled in opposition to HHS's new final rule, finding that constitutional protections against gender and sex discrimination extend to broader issues like transgender healthcare access and discrimination based on sexuality or sexual preference (Jost, 2020). This court ruling, however, has no direct bearing on HHS's final rule, other than to strengthen the potential for future legal challenges it faces (Keith, 2020b). Although the bulk of the controversy surrounds issues of gender, language protections have become collateral casualties in a political debate about the gender identity, reproductive rights, and sexual wellness of patients by mere virtue of their mutual inclusion in a section of federal legislation. The case of Section 1557 highlights several relevant facts: (1) much legislative and judicial activity related to civil rights is essentially unenforceable; (2) protections are liable to change with the ideological vision of incoming administrations; and (3) the securing of civil rights, including linguistic civil rights, is a never-ending and ongoing process to which vigilant attention must be paid.

The Plain Writing Act

Drawing on previous calls to address low health literacy rates by utilizing less legal and medical jargon – i.e., by using "plain language," as opposed to specialized language (Stableford & Mettger, 2007) – in 2010, Congress enacted the Plain Writing Act (Plain Writing Act, 2010). This act outlines specific steps that healthcare providers must take to serve the (written) language needs of all patients. Though not explicitly passed for the benefit of patients labeled LEP, in mandating the use of written medical language that is understandable to the average patient (as opposed to the specialist), the Act increases language protections in general. Some argue that the Act has failed to achieve its stated goals (Stabler, 2013), while others (Koh et al., 2012) insist otherwise. Nonetheless, the Plain Writing Act represents an essential addition to the legal documentation of linguistic civil rights.

Implementation and enforcement of Civil Rights law

The Joint Commission

The primary centralized governing body for healthcare providers in the U.S. is a non-profit organization, formed in 1951, called The Joint Commission (Givan, 2016). The Joint Commission's central function is to certify healthcare providers for receiving federal funds via Medicare and Medicaid reimbursements. Because the federal government mostly implements civil rights protections by controlling federal funding, the Commission plays a significant role in enforcing the Civil Rights Act and related regulations. Since Medicare and Medicaid were introduced in the passing of the Social Security Amendments of 1965, the Joint Commission has administered the only accreditation program recognized by the federal government. Accreditation is voluntary, but no organization will receive federal reimbursements without it, and a significant number of institutions serving LEP patients (especially large hospitals and public health clinics) require federal funds to maintain operations (*ibid.*).

To be compliant with federal Civil Rights law and receive Medicaid and Medicare reimbursements, the Commission requires healthcare providers to establish a variety of quality control measures related to patient care. This includes language rights protections and matters of cultural competence, as stated in the Commission's 2010 publication "Advancing effective communication, cultural competence, and patient- and family centered care: A roadmap for hospitals" (The Joint Commission, 2010). Appendices B and C (pp. 46–63) provide detailed requirements for accreditation based on the linguistic civil rights of patients, and Appendix D (pp. 65–76) outlines the legislative history requiring hospitals to accommodate the communicative needs of patients, with a particular focus on those with vision and hearing impairments.

Even though the Joint Commission has some enforcement power in revoking accreditation, few organizations ever lose accreditation or have significant punitive action taken against them, especially for civil rights violations (Givan, 2016, pp. 96–98; Michael, 1995). Furthermore, providers who do not seek accreditation (generally those who refuse to serve Medicare and Medicaid beneficiaries) are not within the jurisdiction of the Joint Commission and related civil rights guidelines (Reid, 2010). Like EO 13166 and the related departmental guidelines, the Commission ultimately encourages hospitals and other federal aid recipients to self-regulate, something legal and healthcare scholars have criticized for decades (Jost, 1994). As one reviewer of this chapter commented, issues with uneven enforcement raise important questions about the potential for universal language access within profit-driven healthcare delivery systems. The Department of Health and Human Services lists 25 "Enforcement success stories involving persons with limited English proficiency" on their website (U.S. Department of Health and Human Services, 2013). However, because of the many barriers facing LEP patients, the unevenness of enforcement, and the existence of many private providers who do not accept federal funding, the number of cases reported likely lies far below the actual number of incidents.

Legal barriers

Barriers to implementing civil rights protections for patients who speak languages other than English can be characterized in many ways. One larger issue is a lack of explicit legislation directly related to language and health care; another is a lack of enforcement on behalf of the corresponding legislative and judicial bodies (DeCola, 2011). Most of the rights guaranteed to patients are derived from legislative language that refers either to "federal aid recipients" as a collective whole or from interpretations of legislation that arose from court cases dealing with other services, e.g., *Lau v. Nichols* with education. This translates to a weakened infrastructure for implementing protections specifically for patients, which a general lack of resources within U.S. health care exacerbates.

Because language rights guidelines have mostly been interpreted by individual healthcare institutions and the governments of states in which they operate, compliance with Title VI and other regulations varies by location (Khanijou, 2005; Schiaffino et al., 2014, 2016; Youdelman, 2008). In a national survey of language access laws within healthcare institutions, Youdelman (2008) found that 17 states had less than ten requirements regarding language, some of which are states with relatively high LEP populations (e.g., Kansas). California, with over 150 requirements, far outpaced other states. This is likely because, in 1999, California began implementing a series of "threshold language policies," whereby individual agencies determine the proportion of local patients who would have to be monolingual in a language other than English in order for the organization to be responsible for accommodations (McClellan et al., 2012; Snowden & McClellan, 2013). Such policies, in attempting to tailor language access to specific communities, effectively work to deny healthcare access to LEP patients by not accounting for numerically small populations and by leaving open the possibility of manipulating the threshold based on economic concerns.

Practical barriers

Another barrier facing LEP patients in U.S. health care is the low number of bilingual healthcare workers (Brooks et al., 2016; Diamond et al., 2008, 2012; Flores et al., 2003). Because many providers are not themselves bilingual (and even fewer have received the necessary training and certification to provide care in a language other than English), the norm is to rely on a professional interpreter. When a professionally licensed interpreter is unavailable, many healthcare facilities allow patients' family members to interpret or lean on bilingual staff who are not certified to provide interpreting services nor compensated for such services. Flores et al. (2003) found that not only are non-professional interpreters more likely to commit errors but that 63% of errors committed documented in their study had potential clinical consequences (see Chapter 3). The use of non-professional interpreters has been shown to negatively impact outcomes for LEP patients, and although it is forbidden by nearly all guidelines and laws discussed in this chapter, it is nevertheless extremely common within the U.S. healthcare system (Mayo et al., 2016; Nápoles et al., 2010; Tipton & Furmanek, 2016).

Furthermore, Diamond et al. (2012) show that healthcare workers may over- or misrepresent their second-language abilities, and that in part, this stems from utilizing inadequate, proprietary proficiency measurements. After implementing the U.S. Foreign Service's Interagency Language Roundtable Scale, they found that doctors were significantly more likely to downgrade their previously high self-reported proficiency to a lower level. Similar cases have been made for using ACTFL guidelines more consistently (Arocha & Joyce, 2013). In addition to misreporting proficiency, doctors may under-utilize interpreters and interpretation services based on self-reported language proficiency, incorrectly believing their language skills are sufficient to administer care to non-English-speaking patients (Diamond et al., 2008). Even in those interactions where professional interpreters are utilized, because there are no federal- (and few state-level) language requirements to work as an interpreter, the quality of service varies widely within and between different states and individual institutions (DeCola, 2011).[2] Nevertheless, it is important not only that provider and interpreter fluency and other qualifications be accurately reported, but that professional services are utilized when there is language discordance between patient and doctor.

Enforcement and resources for patients

The route a patient must pursue to file a language-related complaint and see action taken on it is complex. As stated above, the main hub of information related to linguistic civil rights as a protected category is the website for the Department of Justice's Working Group on Limited English Proficiency (http://lep.gov). If a patient felt their Title VI language rights had been violated, they could navigate here, find the "Complaints" tab, and encounter a list of 24 federal departments and divisions with whom to file a complaint. If the patient is unsure, they can file their complaint directly with the DOJ's Federal Coordination and Compliance Section, under which the Working Group is housed.

What ultimately happens is that the Office of Civil Rights of the particular federal agency under question (in the case of a health complaint, the Department of Health and Human Services) reviews the complaint and decides whether action must be taken, up to and including revoking federal funds from the offending institution. The patient must file the complaint within 180 days of the alleged incident and must be able to specify which regulations of the Civil Rights Act were violated and how (DeCola, 2011, p. 159). This has resulted in some strengthening of language services via successfully resolved complaints (DeCola, 2011; The Joint Commission, 2010), but in most cases, the lack of available monetary and administrative resources causes a lack of enforcement of language rights guidelines (Khanijou, 2005).

Considering the low level of health literacy in the general population (Sudore et al., 2009) – and among LEP patients specifically (Penaranda et al., 2012) – merely figuring out which agency to contact is itself a daunting task. Accessing the resources to follow through with a legal challenge revolving around civil rights violations in a federally funded healthcare institution is doubly so. However, the likelihood is that a patient would first seek assistance from hospital administrators. In this case, protocol likely varies by institution.

Conclusion

In a society as large and diverse as the modern U.S., language intersects with health care and other services in complex ways. Despite more than half a century of legislative decisions, executive orders, and court cases establishing the parameters of language rights in the U.S., lacking English proficiency still places patients at a disadvantage in the healthcare system, creating health disparities related to ethnolinguistic background. One of the primary goals of many applied linguists working within the field of health care is to address these disparities from a variety of perspectives, using linguistic insights to increase the quality of services rendered by healthcare institutions. This is an ongoing sociocultural and legal process, and much work must still be done to secure equal access to healthcare services and to address language barriers from the patient's perspective (Yearby, 2014, 2015).

Crucial to this goal is increasing **health literacy** among patients (Wynia & Osborn, 2010). As defined in 2000 by HHS, NIH, and the National Library of Medicine, health literacy measures "the degree to which individuals have the capacity to obtain, process, and understand basic health information and services needed to make appropriate health decisions". Therefore, increasing health literacy means increasing awareness of the functions of the healthcare system and the patient's rights within it. It also means addressing the accessibility of the language (both spoken and written) used within health care from the patient's perspective. When a patient's health literacy increases, that patient is better prepared to face a health crisis should one arise, and this will ultimately increase the overall level of care provided to people living in the U.S.

However, health literacy as a "soft skill" is difficult to achieve, especially for those considered LEP within federal or public services (see Chapter 5 for more discussion). The lack of interpreters available in hospitals, for example, is compounded by the lack of high-quality translated material for LEP patients. Fortunately, researchers have shown that several approaches effectively increase health literacy among people with LEP. Soto Mas et al. (2015) advocate a community-based approach that partners patients, healthcare providers, and local educators to spread awareness and increase the availability of translators and interpreters within the medical field.

Applied linguists can play a valuable role in such an approach as facilitators of patient-centered and language-focused research and advocacy. They can mobilize sociolinguistic insights about, for example, the role that language ideologies play in institutional spaces (Carter, 2014), the effects of linguistic discrimination on health disparities, or culture- and language-specific health metaphors and conceptions of healthcare practices (Magaña, 2019). Applied linguists can also work across disciplines to employ the expertise of (and impart an understanding of the importance of sociolinguistic competencies to) medical researchers and practitioners. Such work fosters a new paradigm of language rights and access in health care that is predicated on the needs and strengths of the individuals and groups in question. Investigators working within this type of paradigm can advance research questions about the social dynamics of language while increasing awareness about the language- and health-related issues facing the very individuals with whom they work. The other chapters in this volume are dedicated to outlining this role, but an important first step is understanding the legislative and judicial history of language access in health care, and the divides between policy and practice, or between theory and reality.

Questions and activities

1. Have you or someone you know ever experienced a language barrier when seeking medical care? How does your experience relate to the descriptions in this chapter, especially considering the differences between policy and practice that this chapter highlights?

   If you have not experienced a language barrier, have you or someone you know experienced any other barriers seeking medical care – for example, difficulty following dense medical jargon or descriptions of conditions and treatments? How might that be similar to the barriers described here?
2. Visit a local hospital or health clinic and observe the signage and documents provided. Are languages other than English represented? If so, which ones? Now compare this to ethnic and linguistic demographics for the area, and comment on the concordance (or lack thereof) between the local population and the services provided by healthcare institutions.
3. An undergraduate student majoring in Spanish at Wichita State University started a campaign to encourage Spanish-speaking patients to always request an interpreter to increase the demand for professional interpreters and translators. What are some practical ways you could apply the concepts in this chapter relating to language, health care, and civil rights to help ensure enforcement of Title VI guidelines? How would this be specific to your community?

Notes

1 Though the original language specifies "translators," this is likely meant to refer to both in-person interpreting and written translation.

2 Despite the lack of federal- and state-level proficiency requirements to be employed as a healthcare interpreter, there are programs available, offered by groups such as the Certification Commission for Healthcare Interpreters and the National Council on Interpreting in Healthcare.

3 Language access and interpretation in health care

By the end of this chapter, you will be able to answer these questions:

1. What are *language access and language acceptance?*
2. To what extent do policies and practices for healthcare interpreting and language-concordant care acknowledge and build on patients' language practices and repertoires?
3. To what extent are digital technologies (such as remote interpretation platforms and telehealth) changing our expectations for meaningful language access?
4. What skills and knowledge are needed for interpreters to be qualified to interpret in a particular healthcare context and use the chosen modality?

Introduction

> *Yo quiero expresar mi experiencia, que me sucedió porque estoy en un dilema. [...] Mi hijo sufrió una cirugía de (a)pendicitis. En el primer caso me, me dijeron, en urgencias de [nombre de hospital] no tiene [...] apendicitis, tiene una enfermedad de transmisión venérea...Me lo llevé a mi casa, le dieron el medicamento... a raíz del medicamento, todo el apéndice se le explotó en el estómago. Se le explotó. Llegué otra vez a la clínica a... [...] llegué y me dijo la doctora es de emergencia, tienes que llevarlo porque se le... se le reventó el apéndice [...] Es por lo mismo, porque nosotros no sabemos expresarnos ¿verdad? Por eso pasa esto.*

DOI: 10.4324/9781003041184-3

> I want to share my experience, what happened to me, because I have a dilemma. My son had appendicitis surgery. At first, they told me, in the emergency department at [name of hospital], he doesn't have appendicitis. He has a venereal disease…I took him home, they gave him medicine…because of the medicine, his whole appendix exploded in his stomach. It exploded. I got to the clinic again to…I got there, and the doctor told me that it was an emergency. You have to take him because…his appendix burst…It's because of the same thing, because we don't know how to express ourselves, right? That's why this happens.

This is how Verónica Mireles began her story, standing up to speak to the Latinx families, healthcare providers, interpreters, language researchers, and community organizers at a translingual community meeting in Wichita, Kansas, in early Spring 2020. As the story unfolded, it became clear that a series of miscommunications had occurred due to a lack of professional interpreting services, leading her providers to miss the signs of appendicitis and send her son home without correctly diagnosing his condition. Verónica's story demonstrates how inadequate **language access** services can lead to errors in diagnosis and treatment and, ultimately, adverse health outcomes and heavy financial burdens for speakers of minoritized languages.

When she states that the incident occurred "*porque nosotros no sabemos expresarnos ¿verdad?* (because we don't know how to express ourselves, right?)," Verónica acknowledges that the healthcare system places the burden on her, as a Spanish-speaking immigrant, to describe her own and her family's health conditions, such that the problems resulting from miscommunication cannot be blamed on anyone but herself. This is because of a disposition within the healthcare system toward English as the normal, normative language to be used in public space and a resulting lack of **language acceptance** that fits outside of this norm (Martínez, 2020).

Despite her awareness of the burden the healthcare system places on individuals like her, we know that Verónica has not internalized the responsibility for the medical error because she has taken the initiative to share her story and demand systemic change. Verónica's proclamation of her **testimonio** at the stakeholder meeting was a step forward in the process of **testimonial justice** because she was claiming her right to be heard in an environment in which the participants were likely to believe and support her (Martínez et al., 2021; Showstack et al., 2021). Later, Verónica would share the same story in more public contexts and encourage others to do the same. By telling her story, she was seeking testimonial justice, a right to be heard and believed without prejudice or stereotype (Fricker, 2007), not only within the circle of stakeholders but also in healthcare interactions themselves. For testimonial justice in health care and health equity for Spanish-speaking Latinxs more broadly, the environment within healthcare institutions needs to foster acceptance of diverse language practices and communication needs, and the stories of Spanish-speaking Latinxs need to be heard and listened to. This includes the possibility of voices being raised for legal action when healthcare facilities harm individuals by thwarting federal regulations, an option that was not available to Verónica and her son, as she had chosen to take the burden on herself.

Verónica's son ended up staying at the hospital for a week and a half. Once at home, he could not attend school for another week due to complications associated with the appendix rupture, and Verónica missed work to take care of him. Verónica now faces a medical debt of $85,000. When she filed a complaint with the hospital, she was told that she had signed a document stating that she would not accept financial assistance for the bill. However, nobody had explained this to her before she signed the document, which was only provided in English.

This story depicts the severe consequences that can stem from language barriers in the medical field. If Verónica, who spoke little English, had understood her rights, she would have known to insist that the hospital provide a professional interpreter the first time they visited the emergency department (ED); during that visit, a person who worked at the hospital was eventually sent to interpret, and, according to Verónica, provided inadequate services. Because Verónica was not provided with a qualified interpreter, the first doctor who treated her son made an error in evaluating his symptoms, which led to an adverse outcome that could have been avoided. Even if no interpreter were physically present in the ED, the ED physician should have had the capacity to connect with one on the spot via telephone or video. The major hospitals in Wichita both contract with agencies that provide in-person and remote interpreting services, and therefore, should have the capacity to reach an interpreter at any moment of the day or night.

What happened to Verónica and her son resulted from inadequacies in the language access policies of one hospital, whose state was not enforcing national standards, coupled with limitations on language acceptance in the healthcare system (Martínez, 2020; see Chapter 1 of this volume). As outlined in Chapter 2, the Affordable Care Act's non-discrimination provision stipulates that covered entities are required "to take reasonable steps to provide meaningful access to each individual with limited English proficiency who is eligible to be served or likely to be encountered within the entities' health programs and activities" (U.S. Department of Health and Human Services, 2020a). To meet this requirement, the hospital that Verónica visited with her son contracted with two in-person interpreting companies and also utilized telephonic interpreting when an interpreter was needed immediately. However, in Verónica's case, it appears that these companies were not called, perhaps because hospital staff assumed that she did not need an interpreter because she was responding to medical staff questions in English. Did the staff make a conscious decision not to call an interpreter? Did they feel that communication in English was preferable even though it was clearly not Verónica's preferred language? What did the staff understand about what was needed for effective communication in an emergency care context? Who bears the responsibility of monitoring the provision of language access? How would a less monoglossic English bias have made a difference in the health care outcomes for Verónica and her son? These questions highlight the issues of healthcare language access to be explored in the present chapter.

Verónica told us that although she knew that the communication between her and the healthcare provider was not proceeding well during their first visit to the ED, she did not know that she had a right to request a professional interpreter. According to an interpreter who works on the staff at the hospital where Verónica visited the ED, patients must indicate their language preferences and need for language access services on an intake form that they fill out when checking in. However, hospital staff does not necessarily reference this form when determining whether patients need interpreters. Patients may feel that because they already indicated their need for an interpreter or language-concordant provider on a form, asking for language access services would be inappropriate. This situation exemplifies the need for hospitals and clinics to design **language access plans** that provide them with a framework for deciding whether language access services are needed and how those services should be provided. The process should include a decision about which modality of interpreting (remote vs.

in-person) should be used if language-concordant care is not available. It should also include a way of determining which language is needed so that services are not provided in an inappropriate language (i.e., when a speaker of the Guatemalan indigenous language K'iche', who only speaks rudimentary Spanish, is mistakenly provided with a Spanish interpreter rather than a K'iche' interpreter).

Like Verónica, many of the other stakeholders who participated in a series of community meetings held in Wichita in 2020 and 2021 described situations in which they had not been offered a professional interpreter or had been asked to interpret informally for family members. Many of these individuals were unaware that the healthcare facilities were obligated to provide qualified interpreters or language-concordant providers for patients who needed them. These patients did not have equitable opportunities to attain the highest possible level of health because of language barriers in combination with other circumstances. In addition to language barriers, their health experiences may have also been affected by economic disparities, immigration experience, discrimination based on language and/or race, and the presence of co-morbid conditions such as diabetes and depression. The interactions between these factors can best be understood through a syndemic approach (see Chapter 1), with language access as one important component in supporting individuals with limited English proficiency in attaining the highest possible level of health.

This chapter explores the process of providing language access in health care, the ways that language access can be provided, including through language concordance and different modalities of interpreting, and the professional skills needed for these language access roles.

Process of providing language access

Verónica was a regular patient at a safety-net health clinic that serves the uninsured; the clinic, though not tied to federal guidelines because it did not receive federal funding, usually offered interpretation by bilingual staff or volunteers. However, when leaving the low-income clinic to attend a federally funded healthcare facility for an acute health problem, she faced the most damaging effects of the problems with language access and language acceptance. In the hospital, the bilingual healthcare staff serving as ad-hoc interpreters only appeared when communication difficulties were apparent to the provider. In other moments, Verónica and her son did their best to communicate in English.

One factor that may have contributed to the breakdown in the process of providing language access is that the hospital may not have established an adequate language access plan or an "effective written plan for providing interpreter services that are appropriate to the particular circumstances" (Peña et al., 2019). According to the Center for Medicare & Medicaid Services (CMS), "Language access plans should be tailored to individual organizations, but may include similar sections, such as a needs assessment, language services offered, notices, training for staff, and evaluation…" (p. 2). Additionally, language access plans should include planning for language-concordant care, when possible. Peña et al. (2019) state that the personnel at healthcare facilities should be trained and provided with scripts on the language access services available at the facility. To create a context in which hospital staff consistently value the well-being of patients whose preferred language is not English, language acceptance also has to be prioritized.

The first step in providing language access services is determining that the patient needs assistance. While patients can call a healthcare facility ahead of a visit to request an interpreter, this does not always happen. Therefore, when a patient walks into a facility or attends an appointment without requesting an interpreter in advance, the patient needs to be made aware that interpreting services are available in their language free of charge. At the same time, administrative staff and providers should assess the patient's language needs and determine the best way to provide either language-concordant care or interpreting services, if needed.

Without a fully implemented language access plan, even when staff are making their best effort to address their patients' language needs, procedural errors can be made that lead to inadequate services. For example, a patient may ask to use her child as an interpreter, and administrative staff who wish to appease the patient may fail to inform her of the problems with child language brokering and the availability of professional interpreters. Although **language brokering**, when children serve as interpreters for their parents and other family members, does not always lead to negative emotional outcomes for children, it can cause emotional stress and lead to risky behaviors (Kam & Lazarevic, 2014; López et al., 2019). Another consequence of poorly implemented language access plans is that bilingual healthcare providers may serve as interpreters without proper training and compensation.

Conceptualizing concordance

One ideal situation for Verónica would have been to receive care from **language-concordant providers** or healthcare providers who can communicate effectively in the patient's preferred language. Patients with language-concordant providers display greater trust, show more agreement, and are more likely to follow doctor recommendations, and in some cases have been found to have better health outcomes (Diamond et al., 2012).

However, not just any bilingual healthcare provider is qualified to provide language-concordant care. Diamond and Reuland (2009) argue that a standardized system of reliably describing and reporting physician language proficiency is needed. Without these standardization systems, a physician with a knowledge of medical vocabulary in Spanish and a low level of fluency (or vice versa) could be allowed to communicate with patients like Verónica without an interpreter, potentially leading to miscommunication and/or diminished patient trust. Like most regions in the U.S., few healthcare providers in Kansas speak Spanish proficiently enough and know the specialized vocabulary needed to use the language to communicate with patients in patient care situations without the assistance of an interpreter. This is the case across sectors, including ED, chronic care, clinics, and hospitals; in the ED context, the fact that patients are unlikely to have a prior relationship with providers can increase the potential for negative outcomes due to misdiagnosis. According to Ortega (2018), the problem of physician-patient language discordance with the Spanish-speaking population in the United States should be addressed with a standardized process of Spanish-language-concordant medical education.

On the other hand, the Spanish language skills of bilingual healthcare providers are often classified as inadequate even though these providers possess significant linguistic and cultural capital that is valuable to healthcare interactions (King-Ramírez & Martínez, 2018). According to King-Ramírez and Martínez (2018), there is a need to improve training in a way that recognizes the linguistic and cultural capital of bilingual healthcare professionals and provides them with opportunities to leverage those skills in the facilities in which they work. While bilingual professionals benefit from language training in preparation to serve patients who speak minoritized languages, those professionals who come from the same communities as the patients possess valuable knowledge that they can leverage in their healthcare communication practices.

In the U.S., there are two ways in which bilingual providers can be trained and certified to use a language other than the dominant language in health care. While not standardized across institutions and states, there are particular trainings and exams available for qualified bilingual staff to attain the qualifications of a **dual role interpreter**, and these individuals learn about both language-concordant care and healthcare interpreting; they also learn how to appropriately toggle between the interpreter and provider roles in a way that does not inhibit communication. Alternatively, clinicians can be trained to provide high-quality language-concordant care without the interpreter role. There is a need for increased awareness of these trainings among clinicians and within healthcare institutions, both to avoid the inappropriate use of patients' preferred language by clinicians who are not qualified to provide care in that language and to support the development of local language training programs for clinicians that can improve care for speakers of minoritized languages. The promotion of training and compensation for dual role interpreters and language-concordant providers is a significant step toward avoiding the use of untrained interpreters because bilingual healthcare providers are often asked to interpret or provide language-concordant care even when they are not qualified, which can lead to inequitable care for speakers of minoritized languages.

Ad-hoc interpreters

Healthcare institutions vary widely in their interpretation of what it means to be a qualified interpreter. While healthcare interpreters should ideally be hired professionally and carefully vetted for their qualifications, in reality, interpreting is often provided by **ad-hoc interpreters**, individuals who are not professional interpreters and are called on to interpret specific encounters. For example, bilingual nurses not trained as interpreters left what they were doing at the hospital to interpret for Verónica and the providers who were caring for her son. Ad-hoc interpreters are substantially less reliable for accuracy than professional interpreters; professional interpreters, especially those with higher numbers of training hours, have been found to produce significantly fewer errors than ad-hoc interpreters (Flores et al., 2012).

In addition to unqualified bilingual healthcare providers, ad-hoc interpreters often include patients' family members (and quite often their children). In the stakeholder meeting where Verónica shared her story, a patient named Cecilia also shared the difficulties she experienced when her children had interpreted her healthcare encounters. "Mi dolor es su dolor" ("My pain is their pain"), she said; Cecilia didn't want her grown children to have to hear about her suffering, and it was hard for her to tell the provider about everything she was experiencing when they were there. When Cecilia learned that she had a right to a professional interpreter, she began to use that service regularly.

Modalities of interpreting

In the absence of patient-physician language concordance, a qualified professional interpreter is usually the most appropriate option. This interpreter can be present in the same room as the provider and patient, providing "in-person" interpreting. Some hospitals have in-person interpreters on staff for the most commonly spoken language(s) of the region; others contract with companies that send in-person interpreters when needed. When qualified in-person interpreters are not available, clinics and hospitals can contract with companies that provide remote interpreting services, in which a person in a remote location serves as an interpreter and is accessed via either telephone or tablet. The use of remote interpreters in developed nations is increasing as the presence of immigrants and refugees who are not proficient in the dominant language increases. Reliance on remote interpreting was accelerated during the COVID-19 pandemic due to social distancing recommendations. To decrease the risk of spreading the virus, some healthcare institutions imposed limits on the number of individuals who could be physically present with a patient at a time, which in some cases meant that an in-person interpreter was not permitted. Apart from interpretation for commonly spoken languages like Spanish, remote interpreting services are also a vital resource in care for speakers of less commonly spoken languages because interpreters of such languages are scarce and less likely to be available to provide in-person services.

Healthcare research has compared different interpreting modalities (e.g., in-person vs. remote interpreting) examining their outcomes. The results generally show similarities in interpretation accuracy and patient satisfaction for in-person vs. remote interpreting (although "accuracy" is analyzed differently in literature from different fields) (Crossman et al., 2010).[1] On the other hand, Leemann Price et al. (2012) found that, according to interpreters, interpersonal communication was limited in telephonic interpreting. Drawing from a posthumanist perspective (Barad, 2007; Pennycook, 2018), Martínez et al. (2021) found that Spanish-speaking patients in Ohio tended to miss out on a personal connection with remote interpreters, referring to them as "la máquina" (the machine). For these patients, the use of remote interpreting led to limited conveying of their emotions, made it difficult for the interpreter to explain what was being said in between providers, and led to less negotiation of meaning between the interpreter and the patient. (In Chapter 4, we further explore the processes and impact of the negotiation of meaning in healthcare interactions.)

Martínez et al. (2021) argue that remote interpreting can create an additional layer of separation between the individuals participating in a conversation and can limit the possibilities for communicating about emotions, clarifying the meaning of a speaker's words, and engaging in interpersonal communication. While the significance of the limitations to discursive processes associated with remote interpreting may appear obvious to a scholar of language and interaction, non-linguists are less likely to notice these differences on a conscious level or be able to articulate what is missing from the interaction. There is a need for discursive analysis of interpersonal communication in different interpreting modalities. For example, researchers could compare the types of interactions related to non-clinical topics (i.e., "small talk"), the use of body language, mitigation (linguistic strategies to modify unwelcome effects on a hearer), and epistemic brokering (negotiation of positions of authority) that occur between providers and patients when using in-person vs. remote interpreting, and how those resources are understood in each modality (Allison & Hardin, 2019; Raymond, 2014b).

In addition to remote interpreting for in-person medical encounters, interpreting services can also be provided for telehealth (when a provider visits a patient via a remote service similar to Zoom). The need to provide telehealth services for patients whose preferred language is not English increased in the U.S. during the COVID-19 pandemic, creating an additional challenge to health equity for speakers of minoritized languages. Physicians were not adequately trained to meet patients' language access needs through telehealth (Diamond et al., 2020; Shin et al., 2021), and telehealth platforms did not always include the technology needed for remote interpreting services (Martínez et al., 2020). Even with adequate technology and training, interpreting for telehealth encounters can be challenging when interpreters are not able to see the entire room;

furthermore, during the pandemic there was an added challenge of muffled sound due to the use of personal protective equipment (Shin et al., 2021). Interpreters require specific training and skills to be qualified to provide services in each of the types of encounters mentioned in this section; for telehealth, interpreters must be adept at navigating an online platform with its particular affordances and limitations.

Professionalization of providers and interpreters

Although Flores et al. (2012) and others have demonstrated that a significantly higher proportion of clinically significant errors occur when using ad-hoc interpreters as opposed to trained interpreters, the risk of using untrained interpreters goes far beyond accuracy errors in interpreting. In addition to knowing a context-specific set of vocabulary in Spanish and English and demonstrating an advanced level of fluency in both languages, interpreters are responsible for understanding and applying multiple interpreter roles and adhering to a set of ethical guidelines. For example, basic ethical principles include impartiality and precision of interpreting. Ad-hoc interpreters may violate these principles and thus create confusion by giving the patient information that the health care provider did not state or summarizing what a patient said to the provider and unintentionally leaving out information; a professionally trained interpreter would be expected not to summarize or add information.

In addition to problems with accuracy, using unqualified bilingual healthcare providers as ad-hoc interpreters can lead to increased workload without compensation and a situation in which bilingual staff are pulled away from their other responsibilities at work (Chang et al., 2019; Showstack & Guzman, 2020). Healthcare interpreters are expected to follow a complex code of ethics that recognizes the interpreter's responsibility to serve as a clarifier, cultural broker, and advocate when needed. Still, some scholars have criticized the ethical guidelines put forth by U.S. institutions (e.g., NCIHC) as being overly focused on fidelity and integrity, rather than benevolence and social justice, which are emphasized in ethical guidelines in other fields (King-Ramírez & Martínez, 2018). In addition, Showstack (2021) found that some bicultural Latina interpreters felt limited by their understanding of "professionalism" as represented in the code of ethics, in moments when their intuition and cultural framework pointed toward connecting with the patient on a personal level. The dominant way of representing professionalism in the U.S. could potentially limit space for reflection of cultural values, such as the Hispanic/Latinx values of **personalismo** (supporting interpersonal relationships over institutional ones) and **simpatía** (friendliness), among certain minoritized groups (see Magaña, 2021).

According to Hsieh (2008), a common assumption is that the interpreter's only role is to convey information or to serve as a "conduit" between the provider and the patient. She describes the conduit model as conceptualizing interpreters as robots ("nonthinking, nonfeeling, and yet highly skilled translation machines," p. 1367). However, the interpreter's role goes far beyond simply conveying information. In addition to the **conduit** role, interpreters may also take on the roles of the **clarifier**, who provides specific information in cases when cultural differences create communication barriers; the **cultural broker**, who provides a cultural framework for understanding the message being interpreted; and the **patient advocate**, who acts outside of the bounds of the interpreted interview when she determines that there is a need to advocate for the patient's quality of care. Raymond (2014a, 2014b) shows how interpreters enact various interpreter roles through what he calls "epistemic brokering," which allows them to become socially aligned by negotiating what types of knowledge belong to each participant and rendering speakers' utterances in a way that the listener is more likely to understand; this role can support the development of positive relationships between the patient and the provider.

Interpreter training programs explore ethical standards and the enactment of the interpreter's various roles. In some states, professional healthcare interpreters are required to obtain a certification and/or complete a certain number of hours of training (usually at least 40). In contrast, other states, such as Kansas, have received pressure from advocacy groups to require such training.

Even with a 40-hour training, interpreters may not be prepared to optimize communication with every modality of interpreting and type of healthcare setting. Remote interpreting requires an additional set of knowledge and skills, including different basic protocols and etiquette and particular ways of setting up and utilizing equipment (Cestari et al., in press). In addition to preparing for the interpreter role using a particular modality, healthcare interpreters need to possess ample content knowledge, including technical vocabulary, related to the type of healthcare encounter for which they will be interpreting, and understand the types of questions, diagnoses, and procedures associated with that type of encounter. For instance, interpreting for a routine visit between a provider and patient who already have a relationship will be quite different from interpreting during an emergency situation. Without this knowledge, they may not be prepared to interpret effectively in that particular situation.

As an example, one of Rachel's undergraduate students "Daniela,"[2] a heritage speaker of Spanish, was volunteering as an interpreter at a local women's clinic as part of a service-learning requirement for an advanced Spanish language course. Daniela did not know much about women's pelvic exams before interpreting at the clinic. No one in her family had talked to her about women's health issues; nor did Daniela have first-hand experience with a pelvic exam herself. Daniela was standing between the patient and the doctor when the doctor directed the patient to position herself for the exam. When the patient spread her legs, Daniela immediately felt confused and uncomfortable. Although Daniela did not report difficulties interpreting in other healthcare encounters, she had not been prepared to interpret in this particular context. Clearly, she should not have been asked to interpret in this setting without first learning about the routines associated with typical women's health procedures (or at least after a few shadowing sessions). Daniela's example illustrates that preparing for interpreting encounters is an on-going practice as new interpreters learn to anticipate the content and language expectations for specific healthcare interactions. New interpreters also need support managing the emotional ups and downs when their own knowledge gaps interfere with their sense of professionalism as an interpreter. Applied linguists are able to support the professionalization of interpreters by helping to raise awareness about the interconnectedness of medical knowledge, language proficiency, and contextual schema in interpretation encounters. They can also contribute to the development of partnerships between health clinics and university programs that train interpreters by engaging clinicians and interpreting students in conversations about specific types of healthcare encounters and the communication needs of specific groups of patients.

The professionalization pathway of heritage language learners as interpreters

Even as the professionalization of healthcare interpretation has improved, understanding the experiences and professional development needs of heritage language speakers in this career pathway remains an area in need of greater interchange between applied linguists and healthcare providers. Heritage speakers' family and community language experiences provide them with a unique set of skills and knowledge that can serve as a base for further preparation for careers as healthcare interpreters or language-concordant clinicians (Salgado-Robles & Lamboy, 2019). As they prepare to enter the medical interpreting profession, what kind of pedagogy supports heritage speakers' bilingual repertoire, including knowledge of medical terminology in target languages, while supporting their professional identity as skilled bilingual/bicultural practitioners? How do we productively build on prior experiences they may have had as ad-hoc interpreters, interpreting for their families, often starting at a very young age?

These past experiences can be taken into consideration and incorporated into heritage language curricula for students of all ages, and heritage language learning for the health professions (HLHP) can begin as early as high school, as demonstrated by Glenn's successful medical Spanish program for high school students in McAllen, TX (Martínez, 2020). Martínez and San Martín describe HLHP as

> …a novel approach to language teaching that merges methodological approaches from LSP, HL pedagogy, and CSL to produce advanced, targeted language proficiency and contextualized understanding of the public health issues surrounding the health and health care of Latinos in the United States.
>
> (Martínez & San Martín, 2018, p. 11)

The HLHP model incorporates principles of content-based language learning, direct language instruction that draws on language practices developed in the home/community environment, and critical reflection and analysis.

Rachel has explored community service-learning models as a platform that enables heritage language speakers to reflect on childhood memories of ad-hoc interpreting, often painful and difficult to recall, as they develop their own bicultural/lingual professional identities as interpreters (Showstack, 2019a). For example, in Spring 2022, Latinx students in Rachel's *Practicum in Spanish for the Professions* course shared their *testimonios* about emotionally difficult experiences when they attended medical appointments with a family member, and the healthcare institution did not offer professional interpreting services. One Latinx student, Iván, described interpreting a conversation in which the doctor cited death as one of the possible outcomes of his mother's health condition. As a young adult, Iván had to translate into Spanish the steps his mother needed to follow in order to minimize this risk. Iván recalled feeling unable to interpret in the even tone used by the physician; rather, his words conveyed his emotional distress and fear. Iván concluded this *testimonio* by critiquing the healthcare language policy in Kansas and calling for action to prevent others from experiencing similar traumatic interactions. Iván's *testimonio* was video-recorded and edited for public dissemination at an *Alce su voz* event, on the organization's website, and on social media. Ivan's *testimonio* prompted community members and other students in the *Spanish for the Professions* program to reflect on their own unsettling histories as ad-hoc interpreters and commit to advocating for themselves and others. Applied linguists can continue to explore ways for bilingual students to draw on their own experiences in the process of community engagement around language access, an avenue we will further address in Chapter 6.

Conclusion

In this chapter, we have introduced and explored the concepts of language access and language acceptance, examined the role of healthcare language access policies in supporting health equity, considered our changing expectations for language access in light of emerging digital technologies, and discussed the preparation needed for interpreters to be qualified to interpret in a particular healthcare context using a specific modality.

The opportunity for Verónica to share her experiences at the community meetings was an important first step towards testimonial justice; next, Verónica's story needed to be shared more broadly, and especially with those who were responsible for shaping language access legislation. This sharing was achieved by recording Verónica's testimony on film after the stakeholder meetings and including it in a video later disseminated to Kansas policymakers, ultimately leading to the development of a bill requiring Kansas healthcare institutions to provide qualified interpreters. Verónica wanted other Spanish-speaking Latinx in Kansas to claim opportunities to tell their stories to let state governing bodies and healthcare institutions know about the injustices occurring in Kansas and demand systemic change; there remains much more work yet to be done.

Questions and activities

1 What went "wrong" in the communication about Verónica's son's condition? What additional information would you want to better understand the encounter between Verónica, the ER providers, and her son? How could better language access have affected the outcome of his visit?
2 How does modern technology affect your communication in your healthcare encounters? What is left out of communication using different modalities (e.g., text messages, videoconferencing)? What is added?
3 Find five friends who grew up speaking a language other than English at home and ask each of them whether they have ever interpreted for a family member in a healthcare context. If they have, ask them to describe the context in which they interpreted and how the experience made them feel. What were some of the similarities and differences between your friends' experiences?

Notes

1 The patients' high level of satisfaction indicated on surveys could be related to a phenomenon known as "the ceiling effect," which refers to a notion that this group of patients is likely to rate any language assistance highly. Thus, it is not clear from the literature how patients might be affected by the potential limitations to interpersonal communication in remote interpreting situations.
2 A pseudonym was used to protect the student's anonymity.

4 Language, culture, and power in clinical interactions

By the end of this chapter, you will be able to answer these questions:

1. What are some of the inequalities that language minoritized speakers face in health care?
2. What is the role of cultural humility and competence in doctor-patient consultations?
3. How do clinicians and patients enact power in medical interactions, and how can they share power?
4. What is translanguaging, and how can it impact health-care interactions?

Introduction

> *Yo he tenido experiencias con doctores, como que ahorita últimamente ya na' más lo hacen todo a la carrera. Y ya no quieren, no quieren escuchar. Si le quieres decir algo, "o no tienes que hacer otra cita para eso." No te saben escuchar.*
>
> I have had experiences with doctors, like lately, they just do everything quickly. And they don't want to; they don't want to listen. If you want to tell him something, "oh no, you have to make another appointment for that." They don't know how to listen to you.
>
> (Marta, a woman in her 50s)

When Spanish speakers in rural California were asked what they needed during medical consultations with their doctors, most

DOI: 10.4324/9781003041184-4

said they needed to be *heard*. Marta's statement that her doctors "*no te saben escuchar*" was a common complaint. They explained that doctors and nurses did not give them attention or show interest in what they had to say. Spanish speakers described feeling dehumanized, overlooked, not valued, or as if doctors and nurses were not on their side, all of which suggest they experienced poor communication with healthcare workers (Magaña, 2020).

The structure of the healthcare delivery system in the U.S. means that many patients feel they aren't being heard. Clinicians are typically highly pressed for time as they are pressured to see patients during short appointments because their earnings are affected by the number of patient visits. It is common for primary care doctors to have a 15-minute appointment scheduled for each patient, which negatively impacts the quality of doctor-patient dialogue for both doctors and patients. However, minoritized language speakers are affected disproportionately, creating further healthcare inequalities. For example, they often experience miscommunication with their doctors to the extent that it can result in a barrier to treatment adherence (Hartley & Repede, 2011). Unfortunately, the U.S. healthcare system is not attentive enough to cultural and non-English language orientation considerations, and thus it often fails to meet the needs of language minoritized groups (Showstack et al., 2019).

Research identifies a number of factors in the disproportionate impact of miscommunication on members of language minoritized people. For example, L2 communication anxiety in seeking health care services that goes beyond general L2 communication anxiety is common (Zhao et al., 2021). This anxiety results in language minority patients being less likely to access health care than their English-speaking counterparts (Betancourt et al., 2011; Himmelstein et al., 2021). Racial discrimination by healthcare workers is an unfortunate reality, and many Latinos mistrust doctors and the healthcare system (Cheng et al., 2018; Steinberg et al., 2016). Spanish-speaking Latinos may also have concerns about immigration status, insurance, the financial impact of missing work, among other factors and many are likely to avoid health care as a result (Himmelstein et al., 2021).

Attentiveness to the communication needs of language minority speakers can help address disparities. A language-concordant clinician is perhaps the ideal solution (Ngo-Metzger et al., 2007). A study of Spanish-speaking patients with limited English proficiency showed that seeing doctors who spoke Spanish increased patient compliance with prescribed medication plans, outcomes, and satisfaction with care over interactions with interpretation services (Diamond et al., 2019). One reason may be that interpreters are not familiar with culturally relevant language about prevention and treatment of disease; however, practitioners who speak Spanish may also lack this competence (Ortega & Prada, 2020).

Indeed, linguistically minoritized groups in the U.S. experience disadvantages from the lack of culturally competent clinicians (Cheng et al., 2018; Steinberg et al., 2016). The Association of American Medical Colleges describes three central domains for cultural competence: understanding people's healing traditions and systems; understanding differing values, cultures, and beliefs; and having cross-cultural clinical skills to communicate effectively. Despite efforts to train medical professionals to offer culturally competent and patient-centered care, the preferred approach to the health care of Anglophones is still normalized and imposed onto other minoritized groups. This creates inequities, which culturally competent healthcare workers can remedy.

A study of Spanish-speaking participants in rural California reported on participants' issues with and recommendations for improving healthcare communication, including the need for friendlier and more attentive service, which aligns with Latino cultural constructs (Magaña, 2020). For example, even though clinicians have limited time with their patients, a brief greeting can make a difference for Latino patients, reflecting the value this community places in *simpatía* and *personalismo* (Juckett, 2013). Such a gesture could help mitigate patients' issues with unfriendly encounters and feeling rushed. On the other hand, when clinicians break cultural norms, it hinders communication with Latino patients. These findings highlight the importance of cultural constructs for avoiding interpersonal conflicts in healthcare settings. Demonstrating cultural knowledge not only supports more humane health care but can also empower patients. For example, when Spanish-speaking Mexican patients feel that their doctors understand the challenging experience of being a rural immigrant in the U.S. as well as recognizing the strengths of that community, patients will be more likely to trust the clinician and feel empowered to share their concerns.

Clinicians should have an awareness of healthcare-related cultural constructions within the communities they serve. For instance, among some Mexican-origin communities, *susto* "fright" is a common ailment caused by a profound psychological impact on a person (e.g., seeing a ghost); treatments for mental health issues involve *pláticas,* culturally sensitive heart-to-heart talks (De la Torre & Estrada, 2015). As De la Torre and Estrada point out, healthcare workers can only understand patients' "[e]motional and physiological responses to these perceived illnesses" if they are "both linguistically and culturally aware of these beliefs" (p. 135). Further complicating this task, not all Mexican communities have the same cultural beliefs around ailments and treatment.

Cultural competence should be viewed as an ongoing learning process instead of as expertise or skill that can be mastered because cultural influences can change over time and space (Yeager & Bauer-Wu, 2013). Given human complexity, interventions meant to provide cultural competence should not include overgeneralizations about the behavior and values of people. Not only can people and communities vary, but such generalizations may promote harmful stereotypes. They may also promote a paternalistic approach to health care for patients with cultural perspectives on health that differ from the biomedical approach.

Scholars have proposed **cultural humility** as a necessary corrective to the idea that cultural competence is fixed knowledge. Cultural humility is founded on three principles: lifelong learning, power imbalances, and institutional accountability (Tervalon & Murray-García, 1998). Practicing cultural humility requires a persistent disposition to learn, self-evaluate, and critique. This critical reflection is needed to recognize the power asymmetries that occur in doctor-patient relationships. Through this lens, clinicians are encouraged to be aware of their implicit biases and have openness in learning about others' values and beliefs. Finally, cultural humility is an approach characterized by institutions that hold themselves accountable for generating "mutually beneficial and non-paternalistic partnerships with communities on behalf of individuals and defined populations" (Tervalon & Murray-García, 1998, p. 123). Cultural humility and cultural competence are synergistic and complementary; the first stresses the process (approach), while the latter emphasizes the product (knowledge, which continues to grow) (Stubbe, 2020). Both are crucial in offering **patient-centered care**.

The following sections will explain why understanding illness and well-being from patients' perspectives is critical and how the power dynamics interfere in centering patients' knowledge. Finally, this chapter will introduce the role of translanguaging in health care and offer suggestions for creating more welcoming spaces for language minority speakers living in multilingual contexts.

Power and discourse in patient-doctor interaction

People affected by healthcare barriers are the experts on these issues. Therefore, identifying their knowledge and giving them a voice help shed light on successful interventions and communication (Deeb Sossa, 2019). While advances in medical technology offer cutting-edge biomedical approaches to health care, offering the space to listen to patients attentively leads to a more holistic understanding of their health experiences (Frank, 2013). Unfortunately, for linguistically and culturally minoritized people, who may also face structural inequalities and discrimination, their knowledge about health experiences may be silenced and absent. While Chapter 3 examined the importance of the process of sharing and amplifying the *testimonios* of speakers of minoritized languages in community and public spaces, here we explore the importance of recognizing patients' voices in healthcare encounters.

Centering the voices of affected communities offers solutions in health care, as an ethnographic study by Briggs and Mantini-Briggs (2016) illustrates. This study shows how communication-based inequities in health services exacerbated a mysterious epidemic among an indigenous population in Venezuela who predominantly speak Warao. Ultimately, the mysterious disease took 38 lives, mostly children, starting in 2007. During the epidemic, the parents of the sickened children sought local healers, who referred them to medical doctors. However, doctors and the nurses they employed failed to earn parents' trust, partly because they did not listen attentively to parents' stories or consider them as knowledge producers. They shut down narratives, stressing highly specific questions that demanded short responses, and sought to correlate what they could hear through a stethoscope with the children's parents' statements. The Warao people felt that doctors and nurses portrayed themselves as the only knowledge producers with information about their children's illness. They found this frustrating and therefore returned to traditional healers. Medical personnel, therefore, blamed the Warao community for their health conditions, which further soured trust. Epidemiologists visited the Warao people to investigate the epidemic, and they exhibited similar behaviors to the Westernized doctors and nurses. They interviewed parents of deceased children and local leaders, collected samples (of blood and water), facts (demographic information), and information about symptoms children had exhibited, but did not seek community members' narratives or allow them to ask questions. Recognizing a lack of health/communicative rights, the Warao people became less willing to participate in the investigation. The community members were shocked when these epidemiologists reported that Warao people were "closed nature" and responsible for the children's deaths. Epidemiologists failed to recognize the **health/communicative inequity** that Briggs and Mantini-Briggs's (2016) ethnographic approach identified. Both the doctors and scientists portrayed Spanish as the language of science and modernity, and Warao as the choice of ignorance and superstition (Briggs, 2019).

Wishing to share their narratives, Warao parents and local leaders worked with another team including a medical anthropologist (Charles Briggs), a Venezuelan physician (Clara Mantini-Briggs), and a local healer. In contrast to the previous communication approaches, this team recognized the health/communicative inequities affecting the community and displayed humility and openness by thoroughly listening to parents' narratives and valuing their knowledge. Through those narratives, the group gathered rich details about children's symptoms that led to a rabies diagnosis, solving the mystery and offering solutions to prevent a recurrence of the deadly disease. This case provides evidence of how language and health are fatally entangled for indigenous populations and how centering local knowledge through communicative justice in health can offer solutions.

The medical practitioners who worked with the Warao community failed in part because their medical interviews were not patient-centered. Medical interviews require a physician to have both analytical and interpersonal skills to diagnose patients. While their analytical skills can lead clinicians to diagnostic reasoning, interpersonal skills can lead to establishing rapport with patients and facilitating communication. Fortunately, a patient-centered approach has become more common among doctors and nurses in the U.S., which has offered numerous improvements that encourage clinicians to empower patients, recognizing that, much like the Warao parents, they have the greatest knowledge of their own bodies and experiences. To guide a medical interview using a patient-centered approach, doctors and nurses are expected to (a) understand the patient's psychological and social context, (b) build a therapeutic relationship, and (c) educate the patient (Heritage & Maynard, 2011). Building such a relationship with patients in a medical interview is particularly essential since patients may be expected to reveal very personal and sensitive information about themselves and their families to a clinician they may have just met.

Unfortunately, some clinicians do not have adequate interpersonal skills to implement their training, and this leads to miscommunication and medical errors (Lang, 2012). One of the reasons for poor communication is the asymmetrical power relationship between doctor and patients. Language and communication-based studies devoted to analyzing doctor-patient interactions or patient experiences during medical interviews demonstrate the impact of power imbalances (Ainsworth-Vaughn, 1998; Cordella, 2004). There is evidence that educating practitioners about how these power differences function at the discourse level can have implications for improving communication between doctors/nurses and patients, ultimately leading to better patient outcomes (Lang, 2012).

The causes of power asymmetry between doctors/nurses and patients include differences in socioeconomic status, clinicians' specialized medical knowledge, patients' constructing the authority of the clinician, patients' vulnerability due to feeling ill or uncomfortable in healthcare settings, as well as other social inequalities. A U.S. study shows that Whites are more likely to be on a first-name basis with their doctors than patients of color, suggesting that race and ethnicity play a role in asymmetry among English-speaking Americans (Ainsworth-Vaughn, 1998).[1] Closing the gap with clinic patients, who typically have fewer financial resources, may be more complicated than closing the gap with private practice patients. The long-term relationship that a private practice patient has can also build trust that makes power asymmetry less impactful.

A community-based study on women of color's experiences with their clinicians while seeking care during their pregnancy and birth identified disparities according to race (Altman et al., 2019). The study revealed that doctors share more health information with patients they perceive as White, having higher education, and having higher social status. They also spend more time with these patients and build a stronger rapport. For example, they are more likely to offer information about themselves, which can make patients feel closer to them. Most of the women of color who participated in the study experienced "[l]ack of information exchange, or incomplete information" (p. 3). As a result, they felt "uncertain and confused, fearful, left out of decision making, and disrespected and violated, all [of which led] to the feeling of not being valued or cared about" (p. 3).

One of the participants in Altman et al.'s study shared a traumatic birth experience that was exacerbated by a lack of information from the doctors and nurses who treated her. Her uterus ruptured during labor, and she had an emergency cesarean birth. She reported being confused about what having a ruptured uterus meant throughout the experience. She sought explanations from her doctor, but she was not offered the information she needed to understand what had happened to her, its implications, or the surgery she was undergoing. She felt not cared for, not valued, and not deserving of knowledge. Like other women in the study, she felt disempowered due to her doctor's failure to treat her with respect or as a person of value. This mistreatment is a heavy burden to bear when someone has survived a physically and emotionally traumatizing event. Failing to communicate knowledge that these women deserved to know made it impossible for them to trust their doctors.

Applied linguistics studies have shed light on other ways in which discourse evidences power dynamics. In a medical interaction, methods of claiming power include interruptions, posing questions, and speaking at length (Ainsworth-Vaughn, 1998). Interruptions are a sign of power because they challenge a speaker's right to finish their thought. Research has shown that doctors interrupt patients more frequently than patients interrupt doctors (Magaña, 2021). Medical interpreters also interrupt patients more often than they interrupt physicians (Davidson, 2014). As well as a sign of claiming power, interruptions in healthcare interactions can be dangerous. In analyzing the discourse of emergency department patients, Slade et al. (2008) found that the interruptions of clinicians led to fragmented stories, missing information, and delayed diagnosis. Clinicians who did not interrupt their patients generated a feeling of ease conducive to good patient care. Erzinger's (1991) examination of a medical interview between a Hispanic patient and a doctor who spoke Spanish as a second language shows that because the doctor did not interrupt the patient, the interview had fewer awkward or clumsy interactional features than interactions in which doctors had interrupted more often. Asking a question is also a power move because speakers who pose a question claim the right to choose the next speaker, the topic, and the progression of the conversation (Ainsworth-Vaughn, 1998). Studies have shown that patients typically ask very few questions (Cordella, 2004; Frankel, 1990). However, racial and ethnic minoritized group members ask fewer questions than non-Hispanic White patients (Ainsworth-Vaughn, 1998; Magaña, 2021).

When doctors use medical jargon with patients without explaining the terms, they can exacerbate the asymmetry between them and their patients. Using medical jargon can compromise patients' health since patients may not seek clarification. Some practitioners do not greet their patients, and some speak of their patients, even in their presence, in the third person (e.g., when addressing another doctor). This is a distant style of communicating with patients; such distance is a way to objectify patients and deny them a balanced relationship (Wodak, 1996).

Empowering patients entails minimizing interruptions; using informal language, lay terms, or colloquialisms; and engaging patients in small talk to create a more interpersonal relationship (Magaña, 2021). Yeager and Bauer-Wu (2013) remind us that healthcare workers must consider the privilege and power of their profession and its effect when communicating with patients. They suggest the need to practice humility to lessen power imbalances and share power with patients. This might mean creating a space for them to speak and ask questions to be fully informed and engaged in healthcare decisions in an actual interaction. Simply asking a patient, "Do you have any questions?" does not suffice. Doctors/nurses must create a welcoming environment through friendliness, approachability, creating a human connection with patients, making small talk, self-disclosure, etc. The following section will delve into what it means to create a welcoming space that fully *accepts* patients and their languages in the discussion on translanguaging in health care.

Transcultural competence and translanguaging in health care

Applied linguists have devoted significant efforts to exploring cultural competence in teaching language and culture to second language learners. When cultural competence is viewed as a (native) speaker's ability to engage with another culture, where communities are perceived as being bounded geographically under nationalist ideologies, the concept overlooks multilinguals' complexity in how they "interpret, negotiate, and resist different cultural categories" (Lee & Canagarajah, 2019, p. 16). Scholars have proposed **transcultural competence** as a way to capture the complex experience of speakers in multilingual contexts. Transcultural competence transcends fixed categories and boundaries around essentialized culture. The prefix "trans," here, emphasizes that communication constantly transforms established norms and associations with a language (Canagarajah, 2013; Pennycook, 2007). It represents the complex experiences of minoritized language speakers in multilingual contexts who may have a range of exposure to and influences on the dominant culture and language. In U.S. healthcare settings, transcultural communication with Latinos may require familiarity with patients' socialization practices, meaning knowledge of their social, linguistic, and cultural systems and the issues marginalized groups in the U.S. face concerning language, power, and society (Martínez, 2010; Martínez & Schwartz, 2012).

Translanguaging is a way to account for the complex language practices of multilingual speakers. As Garcia and Wei explain, it is "the speakers' construction and use of original and complex interrelated discursive practices that cannot be easily assigned to one or another traditional definition of a language but that make up the speakers' complete language repertoire" (García & Wei, 2014, p. 24). A translanguaging lens considers communication to be a unified collection of linguistic features in the speakers' languages "without regard for watchful adherence to the socially and politically defined boundaries of named (and usually national and state) languages" (Otheguy et al., 2015, p. 283). Therefore, it is a more holistic approach to understanding speakers' linguistic repertoires than **code-switching** (i.e., language alternation where languages are seen as separate from each other). Unfortunately, multilingual speakers' practices are often misunderstood, disparaged, and not welcomed in formal spaces such as language classrooms, textbooks, and medical encounters.

Recognizing the role of prestige around language and having cultural humility to adapt to the language varieties (i.e., distinctive form of a language) of locals, even when it means going against standard language norms, can lead to enhanced communication. In her study, Bloom-Pojar (2018) shows that traditional medical Spanish did not necessarily equip a group of U.S. medical volunteers to communicate with rural patients in the Dominican Republic. The U.S. volunteers worked with *ayudantes,* local Dominican helpers, to learn and use patients' local rural Dominican Spanish. For example, U.S. practitioners adopted "Dominicanisms" in their speech and adapted the medical intake forms to reflect the local variety. This process involved translanguaging and resulted in improved communication with the patients and developing relationships with them.

A study of doctor-patient interactions in Spanish provides an illustration of transcultural competence and translanguaging in health care (Magaña, 2021). Dr. Ortiz, a doctor of Mexican origin, adapted his questions to accommodate patients' varieties during medical interviews. He was always attentive to whether patients understood key medical terms or phrases and was strategic in guiding patients to answer his questions. He did this by using colloquialisms, switching to informal registers, and translanguaging with bilingual patients, even though he was newly immigrated to the U.S. and did not grow up bilingual.

Dr. Ortiz's consultation with Alejandro, a Mexican-American patient in his mid-30s who was having anxiety and panic attacks, included numerous switches into English even though the consultation was predominantly in Spanish. At one point in the interview, Dr. Ortiz asked Alejandro whether he had faced situations that trigger a panic attack, such as being surrounded by a crowd. The patient said that when he went out with his roommates, he felt panic. As he started to explain why, he paused. Picking up on his hesitation, Dr. Ortiz switched to English. He asked, "looking at you?" Alejandro was then able to continue, to explain that he felt that others both looked at him and criticized him.

Excerpt from mental health consultation with a male patient (mid-30s)

DR. ORTIZ: ¿Te sientes ansioso o inquieto en lugares o en situaciones en las cuales pudieras tener un ataque de pánico o síntomas relacionados al pánico o donde conseguir ayuda o escapar resulte difícil? Por ejemplo, estar entre mucha gente.

[Do you feel anxious or restless in places or situations where you might have a panic attack or panic-related symptoms or where getting help or escape is difficult? For example, being among many people.]

ALEJANDRO: *Como, hay veces que estamos en mi casa con mis* roommates. *Estamos afuera y nos vamos – a mí en veces me da – me da* panic *porque pienso que me están –*

[Like, there are times when we are at my house with my roommates. We're out, we leave – sometimes it makes me – it makes me panic because I think they are–]

DR. ORTIZ: Looking at you?

ALEJANDRO: Looking at me or criticizing me, *pero no – no – puedo irme.*

[Looking at me or criticizing me, but no – no – I can't leave.]

By engaging in translanguaging practices, the doctor guided the patient to share his feelings. Thus he fostered a welcoming space for bilingual patients by signaling to them that their language practices were valid. He reflected a view that opposes dominant language ideologies: for instance, that bilingualism is seen as a strength for majority language speakers and as a weakness for language minority speakers. Not only is Dr. Ortiz likely less comfortable with translanguaging practices because he grew up in Mexico City, a Spanish-dominant context, but translanguaging deviates from standard Spanish norms and is even disparaged in monolingual contexts. Thus his choice is highly deliberate, reflecting his patient-centered approach.

Dr. Ortiz was intentional about communicating that he *accepts* patients and their use of language(s) throughout his interviews, as he confirmed during an interview (Magaña, 2021). He was deliberate about centering their voices; for example, when patients used a non-standard word or phrase (*agüidatado, me dio un bajón*), he used that term over the standard medical one (*tristeza, depresión*). Similarly, when patients used terms in English, he recycled their terms. In the following excerpt from the same interaction with Alejandro, Dr. Ortiz summarized the patient's mental health issues using the patient's terminology (*social anxiety*) instead of its Spanish translation.

DR. ORTIZ: OK. Poca depresión, ansiedad y esto que es como *social anxiety*.

[OK. A little depression, anxiety, and this that is like social anxiety.]

Using patients' terms signals both language acceptance and that a doctor is attentively listening (Martínez, 2020). As Martínez (2010) points out, public health workers traditionally frame measures to surmount language barriers as "language assistance," but acceptance of patients' language needs is far more likely to produce effective results than viewing those needs as a problem. In Dr. Ortiz's case, it builds a connection between doctor and patient that facilitates patient care. Healthcare workers should demonstrate language acceptance through awareness of the language varieties of their patients or the willingness to learn and adapt to the variety of patients to avoid making inferiority/superiority distinctions between varieties. This requires cultural humility. Dr. Ortiz is, like many of his patients, of Mexican origin. But given his class status and his experience as a recent immigrant, he is not a part of their community and thus does not speak the local dialect of Spanish as his native tongue. Yet he is conscious of the local language and willing to adapt to it in his interviews as a mode of communication equally valid as his own.

When considering Latino communities, it is also critical to consider non-Spanish-speaking groups; for example, those who speak an indigenous language experience severe issues around language access. In the central valley of California, where these medical interviews in the examples above were conducted, many indigenous people from Mexico do not speak Spanish as their first language; they speak Zapoteco or Mixteco languages, spoken in Oaxaca, Mexico. A reflection of the local languages and varieties spoken in specific regions is essential in medical education to create more inclusive and equitable health care for language minoritized groups.

Conclusion

To summarize, language discordance directly impacts people's healthcare outcomes and contributes to health disparities. This is a social justice issue because it impacts communities of color disproportionately. For example, adults with limited English proficiency underuse medical services for numerous reasons, including mistrust of the medical system, previous experiences with frustration navigating health care, and fear of discrimination. For minoritized language speakers, including those who are bilingual but speak and identify culturally with a minorized language, being in an institutional setting where their heritage language is not *accepted* and their culture is not recognized or respected exacerbates these gaps. In the U.S., where the Latino population continues to grow, it is crucial to continue addressing these language inequalities.

Increasing the number of multilingual doctors and nurses with transcultural competence can help mitigate disparities. As shown in this chapter, studies that examine the outcomes of culturally relevant and language-concordant health communication between clinicians and patients reveal more positive results for language minoritized people. Cultural competence emphasizes awareness, knowledge, skill, desire, and encounters regarding the target culture. For instance, clinicians will emphasize both friendliness and professionalism during their consultations with Latino patients, who may expect friendliness in line with their cultural values. This approach to cultural competence is synergistic with cultural humility, where the former is the product and the latter the process. Cultural humility is an approach to lifelong learning given the complexity of cultural influences. In contrast, cultural competence highlights the importance of understanding other perspectives on health care beyond Westernized approaches, which can change and fluctuate over time. Practicing cultural humility is crucial for healthcare workers to understand the illness experiences of other cultures.

As discussed in this chapter, cultural humility and competence are essential if all people are to receive patient-centered care. Clinicians must center patients' voices, especially those that are marginalized or silenced, and create welcoming and comfortable spaces to listen attentively. Authentically listening to people can lead to measurably more effective solutions to health concerns. Briggs and Mantini-Briggs's (2016) narrative of offering an indigenous community communicative justice in health by listening respectfully to parents' stories reveals the power of these approaches to care: it led to uncovering the cause of a previously mysterious health epidemic and significant changes to ensure that rabies never runs rampant through that community again.

It is crucial that healthcare workers, public health interveners/policy advocates, and researchers listen to people's feedback on their communication experiences in the healthcare system and how they can be improved (Martínez et al., 2021). The study we previously mentioned on women of color's experiences uncovered that they wanted a connection with their clinicians and that they wanted to feel valued, acknowledged, and respected through information sharing (Altman et al., 2019). Forming a connection between clinicians and patients is crucial so that patients can feel comfortable sharing health-related information with the doctor without feeling judged. For these reasons, an interpersonal connection between doctors and patients can affect patients' health outcomes. Applied linguistics research is particularly fruitful in understanding the different ways in which an interpersonal connection can take place in real-time as well as opportunities that clinicians miss in building rapport.

This chapter overviewed how research in applied linguistics has revealed language-level details of how doctors' and patients' roles are non-reciprocal, indicating unequal power relations. Clinicians must also understand their positions in terms of power and privilege. Power unfolds in specific ways during medical interactions based on who controls the agenda, how information is shared or omitted, question asking, and interruptions (among other factors). Awareness of these power dynamics and working towards mitigating them by empowering patients can lead to enhanced communication with patients. These power differences and language choices made during interactions affect the connection between medical personnel and patients.

As applied linguistics research shows, differences in a patient's and a doctor's socioeconomic background can pose a barrier to communication and forming a connection. Critical reflection on language use, meaning attentiveness to patients' language practices and how people might feel most comfortable sharing information can set a more comfortable atmosphere for patients. An example of this was illustrated when Dr. Ortiz noticed a bilingual patient's hesitation and engaged in translanguaging, mirroring his patient's language practice. The doctor co-constructed the interviews by using his total speech repertoire, translanguaging between formal and informal registers of Spanish, and using English when it is useful. Through his language choices, he demonstrated that he is open to the language practices of others. Indeed, translanguaging is about forming connections with people.

In medical education, it is critical to focus more on how medical personnel can best reach their patients and gain their trust, especially when they come from marginalized communities (Ortega & Prada, 2020). Medical Spanish courses often emphasize technical language but should also address how to connect interpersonally with patients. Practitioners should be aware that Spanish that is too formal can serve to create barriers instead of offering a comfortable communication environment (Ortega et al., 2020). Courses designed to teach medical Spanish should reflect and adapt to the language practices of the communities they serve. Prioritizing local knowledge of communities being served in health care can lead to improving patient-centered care. A richer awareness of the role of language in health care is a step toward achieving this.

This chapter has emphasized why reflecting on clinicians' language choices in healthcare interactions can lead to enhanced communication. This language awareness is particularly valuable in an era when doctor-patient time is limited. Given its impact on outcomes, it will have a strong return on investment in terms of serving an increasingly diverse nation.

Questions and activities

1 What communication skills do language-concordant doctors and nurses need to offer patient-centered care?
2 Think of interruptions in your daily life. How do interruptions differ between peers (friends) and people with different positions of power (instructor/student, doctor/patient)?
3 Consider the following excerpt from a mental health interview between Dr. Ortiz and Érica, a Latina woman in her mid-30s, who deals with depression. How does the doctor claim power? How does the patient claim power?

DR. ORTIZ: ¿Cómo es la depresión? *¿**Como** tristeza o **como** vacío? ¿Cómo?*

What is the depression like? Like sadness or like emptiness? How?

Érica (#20): *Eh, yo no sé qué será vacío, pero yo siento **como** que mi estómago me brinca mucho y **como** que me tiembla....* Um, I don't know what emptiness is like, but I feel that my stomach twitches and trembles.

DR. ORTIZ: hmm [nods]

ÉRICA: *Mucho dolor de cabeza...* Very painful headaches

DR. ORTIZ: Hmm [nods]

ÉRICA: *A veces me siento **como** bien aguados mis pies.*

Sometimes I feel my legs are like jello.

DR. ORTIZ: Hmm [nods], ¿Como *débil?* Like weak?

ÉRICA: *Sí. Y, este, incluso, nomás quiero estar acostada. No salgo nada. No tengo ganas. La mera verdad, me da hasta pena decirle, no tengo ganas ni de bañarme.*

Yes. And, in fact, sometimes I just want to be in bed all day. I don't go out at all. I don't feel like it. The truth is, I even feel embarrassed to tell you, but sometimes I don't even feel like bathing.

DR. ORTIZ: *hmm* [nods]

ÉRICA: *Es una cosa bien horrible.* / It's a very horrible thing.

(Magaña, 2021)

Now reflect on cross-cultural differences in how speakers from other cultures talk about depression. Compare examples from English (e.g., *feeling down, feeling blue, feeling empty*) and another language.

Note

1 It is crucial to note that the formality of language has different implications across cultures. Using titles and last names may not index distance or power asymmetry in the same way in other communities.

5 Language, health, and learning in adult English classrooms

By the end of this chapter, you will be able to answer these questions:

1. How is an adult English language teacher's pedagogical expertise an important resource in efforts to improve health outcomes for linguistically minoritized communities?
2. How is today's healthcare system placing new demands on what contextualized instruction should look like in adult English language classrooms?
3. How have concerns about "low health literacy levels" in the U.S. increased attention to the adult English/literacy education system in health disparities work?

> Sometimes it feels like we're digging with a teaspoon in the desert. Change happens slowly and our efforts may seem small in relation to the enormity of the issues facing students (...) it's important to keep in mind that literacy work is only one front in a larger struggle, and, by itself, it isn't a solution. It will be most effective when it is connected to this larger context rather than seen as a self-contained endeavor, or goal in itself.
>
> (Andy Nash, cited in Auerbach, 1992, p. 130)

Introduction

While the people who use and work in our U.S. healthcare system are linguistically diverse, the system itself is made up of services and

DOI: 10.4324/9781003041184-5

programs that predominantly operate in English. For many adults from immigrant and refugee backgrounds, the ability to speak, be understood and understand others in English is critical to their ability to access care and make informed decisions about their own and their families' health care. In the current socio-political climate in the U.S., public discourse tends to frame "learning English" as a requirement for successful integration and participation in today's healthcare system. Decades of research documenting the link between "limited English proficiency" and poor healthcare access and utilization has, no doubt, reinforced the assumption that good health in the U.S. is tied to one's motivation and success in learning English. Throughout this book, we have discussed the health disparities affecting linguistically minoritized communities who need language assistance in healthcare settings. In this chapter, we explicitly address learners' motivation to learn English as a means to exert greater control over their health care. Our focus on the learning that takes place in classrooms for **adult English language learners (ELLs)**[1] around everyday healthcare experiences should offer an important counterweight to a deficit perspective that depicts learners as lacking in resources, knowledge, and skills.

The U.S. adult ELL population is served by "a patchwork of departments and services, each with its own regulations and requirements" (Wrigley, 2008, p. 170). In 2018, nearly half (43%) of the approximately 1.1 million adult learners served by the U.S. publicly funded adult education system were enrolled in English language programs (U.S. Department of Education, 2021); this number does not include thousands of learners enrolled in community-based programs funded through other streams. The diverse ELL population includes immigrants, refugees, parents, the elderly, "working poor" adults (those under-employed or seeking work), and youth who have aged out of the K-12 system. An increasing number of learners in the system include adults who have not learned to read or write in any language and/or have experienced little or interrupted formal schooling (Bigelow & Vinogradov, 2011).

Questions about how adult ELLs learn new skills are central to any action plan to improve health outcomes for linguistically minoritized communities. There are questions about the widening array of skills required by today's healthcare system, including listening, speaking, reading, and writing in English; print and digital literacy skills; along with critical thinking, problem-solving, and self-advocacy skills needed to be an informed decision-maker about one's health. There are also questions about which skills matter most to learners themselves, which no doubt shift over the lifespan and reflect their health circumstances.

Helping learners make sense of health information can be a daunting task when so much of the information we encounter is not well designed or written. Healthcare tasks have become increasingly bureaucratic – which you may already realize if you have had to decipher a medical bill, read through a health insurance plan, or find a COVID-19 vaccination appointment. Moreover, the **infodemic** – the vast amount of health information about COVID-19 swirling around us, such as health guidelines, risk messages, study findings, data visuals, breaking news, myths, misinformation, and so forth (Naaem & Bhatti, 2020) – taxes everyone's ability to assess what's accurate or trustworthy, even for those who consider themselves educated readers and proficient speakers of English. Managing healthcare tasks, like scheduling an appointment or checking test results, now requires competence with digital devices and platforms that are not standardized across healthcare sectors or providers (insurance companies, safety net systems), and, in many cases, were developed only with dominant English-speaking populations in mind. How are teachers expected to unpack these new demands into accessible, digestible learning chunks (cf. Cromley, 2000) so that learners can connect new information with what they already know? How do teachers work to ensure that classroom activities make a real difference in their learners' ability to navigate our healthcare system?

Particularly inspiring is that adult ESL educators *continue* to pursue answers to these questions, despite the fact that, as reflected in our opening quotation, the work often feels akin to "digging with a teaspoon in the desert." Even though language is widely recognized as a social determinant of health (see Chapter 1), there remains relatively little investment in cross-disciplinary interchange between adult language educators and public health practitioners (e.g., Hohn, et al., 2019; Leong & Santos, 2019; McKinney & Santos, 2019). There are few professional development opportunities or incentives for educators to explore their practice and links to health equity (e.g., Chervin, et al., 2012); the pedagogical wisdom that educators have garnered from teaching their learners to navigate healthcare systems rarely gets disseminated via journals or at conferences. Much of the work educators invest in cultivating partnerships with local healthcare services and providers goes uncompensated and under-recognized. As captured in our opening quotation, the work of adult ELL classrooms must be viewed as "only one front in a larger struggle" (Auerbach, 1992, p. 130) to improve health outcomes for linguistically diverse communities. This chapter offers guidance to readers who wish to see classrooms elevated as a legitimate, valued front in the fight for health equity.

With those goals in mind, this chapter is organized around areas of pedagogical expertise that merit more attention as resources in health equity work. We review a well-established pedagogical approach, **contextualized pedagogy**, and a related concept, **scaffolding**, to explore why skilled educators are vital to broader efforts to support increased access to and participation in our healthcare system. We consider new challenges and opportunities facing adult ELL programs given the increasing complexity of our U.S. healthcare system. We also highlight concerns about "low **health literacy** levels" in the U.S. that have brought important attention to the role of adult ELL/literacy education in health disparities work. Lastly, we take a closer look at group work in beginning-level ELL classrooms to highlight the importance of **talk** and **interaction** in promoting learner engagement with healthcare themes.

Teaching English in the health context: The practice and promise of contextualized instruction

For many decades, integrating health content into the adult ELL curriculum has been a popular choice for implementing **contextualized instruction**,[2] an approach that aims to "[build] content knowledge while simultaneously integrating instruction in – and practice with reading and writing skills, math skills, language acquisition, and soft skills" (U.S. Department of Education, n.d.). Research has shown that quality contextualized learning helps learners see the relevance of instructional activities and transfer new skills and practices to real-world use (Condelli & Wrigley, 2006; Parrish, 2019; Reder, 2013).

We can summarize the value of contextualized instruction around health content in this way:

- Learners learn both English language skills and health content. There is no trade-off between language and content if learners are taught English in the context of healthcare tasks that learners care about (Hohn, et al., 2019).
- Learners practice English by engaging with authentic materials and tasks, meaning that they learn new skills that one would be expected to use in real-world healthcare settings (see Jacobson

et al., 2003). The teacher will emphasize meaningful iterative practice to reinforce learner comprehension and confidence.

- When language learning is connected to a problem or question learners want to solve, they are able to direct the learning process (Wallerstein & Auerbach, 2004). Collaborative problem-solving invites all learners to contribute, regardless of their proficiency level.

Problem-based (Jacobson, 2003) or project-based approaches (Wrigley & Guth, 1992) also provide a productive way to contextualize learning around health topics, as illustrated here:

> **Problem-based learning**. Learners are presented with a story told through the voice of a Mexican-American mother who is worried about cooking with traditional clay pots because she heard they might contain lead: *I talk to my husband, and I tell him not to feed this type of food to our child because it will harm him. And he says, 'What harm? We were all raised like that, eating out of clay pots.'* What should the mother do? The learners look at public health guidelines and invite a public health expert to talk about lead poisoning and other sources of toxic risk in our everyday environments. Learners work in groups to identify different solutions and resources that would be helpful to the family in the story. The learners write short role-plays – in English and Spanish – depicting different decisions that the family might make about eating or not eating out of clay pots.
> (Santos et al., 2011)

> **Project-based learning.** Learners focus on the question, "What are everyday poisons in our households and communities? What can we do to stay safe?" The learners work with their English teacher and a public health expert, who attends several weeks of class, to look at various resources (e.g., bilingual public health posters, lead prevention programs, tenant rights). The learners compile a bilingual resource list that can be shared with other English classes and a checklist of important questions to ask if they are worried about an environmental hazard.
> (Handley et al., 2009)

An important factor in health-contextualized language pedagogy is the teacher's ability to unpack the healthcare context into meaningful learning experiences that, in turn, support real-world applications. What does this unpacking entail? First, teachers need to discern which healthcare tasks are important to address and then identify the array of skills and practices needed to carry out those tasks. Well-trained teachers are particularly savvy at breaking down a task into smaller tasks that can help learners feel more confident in their skills. For example, a teacher can break down the task of making a doctor's appointment into smaller tasks, such as practicing vocabulary for describing different kinds of appointments (e.g., *urgent care, routine check-up*); learning to log into a patient portal; learning to exercise one's right to an interpreter, and so forth. Teachers know that ELL learners need opportunities to practice each of these smaller tasks and apply all that they have learned to actually making a doctor's appointment.

Second, this unpacking means that teachers need to know how to support both content and language learning. The concept of **pedagogical scaffolding** (Wood et al., 1976), a hallmark of Lev Vygotsky's social constructivist theories, is relevant here. This concept emphasizes the primacy of social interaction in the **Zone of Proximal Development** (ZPD), referring to learning opportunities that emerge when a learner is assisted by a more skilled person (i.e., the teacher or a more advanced peer) and thus enable the learner to accomplish more than what she could do on her own. A literal scaffolding in construction work is a temporary structure that supports building. Wood et al. (1976) used this metaphor to explain why learners need social support structures to gain new skills and knowledge. Pedagogical scaffolds are not fixed. Rather, learning involves an ongoing adjustment of the kinds of social support that a learner needs to carry out a task as their confidence and competence grow.

Teachers can support scaffolding in three spheres of activity (cf., Walqui, 2006), as illustrated here:

> *Scaffolding sphere 1*: The teacher plans a curricular sequence that supports the learning of a variety of skills and knowledge related to a particular healthcare context. For example, the teacher engages the learners in a central problem, *What do we do to stay safe at work?* This problem is used to plan classroom activities and set learning goals.
>
> *Scaffolding sphere 2*: The teacher thinks about how she will organize a particular activity (e.g., a role-play activity in which learners practice asking their boss for personal protective

equipment) that supports participation of learners at different skill levels.

Scaffolding sphere 3: The teacher monitors what kind of support learners might need, from moment to moment, as they carry out the role-play activity. How quickly did the learners become comfortable with the language, or do they need more practice? During role-play, do learners introduce new ideas that offer opportunities for future learning?

Experienced language teachers will recognize that these spheres are rarely implemented in lockstep fashion, or as Walqui (2006) observes, "pedagogical action is always a blend of the planned and the improvised, the predicted and the unpredictable, routine and innovation" (p. 164). The adult educator thus can bring expert attention to the learning structures and processes that make new health navigation skills possible.

Along with Walqui (2006), we recognize the value of "bottom-up change" in learning, i.e., when classroom interactions in sphere 3 can make a difference in the scaffolding that occurs in sphere 1. For example, suppose learners learn a new phrase like *informed consent* (sphere 3), and this vocabulary learning invites curiosity, prompts first language translations, and opens up sharing of consent experiences (spheres 2 and 3). This exchange of information, in turn, may prompt the learners to adjust their language learning goals related to patient rights and informed decision-making (sphere 1). Often what aids movement across spheres is the active comparing and contrasting of what learners know with what they learn from others; these interactions can help to restructure the learners' understanding of how the healthcare system works, what their choices are, and what constraints are placed upon them. This knowledge is what we hope learners retain for future use in a real-world healthcare situation.

The expertise involved in this pedagogical unpacking remains poorly understood outside the field of adult education. This scaffolding pedagogy and impact on learners' healthcare decision-making should be part of the knowledge base that links education, language, and health outcomes. However, teachers and learners rarely have the opportunity to share their teaching and learning experiences with health professionals. Nor is the pedagogical expertise of teachers widely recognized as a resource for responding to the learning needs of linguistically minoritized communities in the

U.S. healthcare system. This knowledge also must be shared with medical providers who wish to support their patients' language needs and improve their own communication skills.

Health-contextualizing pedagogy and teacher capacity

While contextualized pedagogy is a practice many teachers value, it promises no magical panacea to the many serious health inequities facing linguistically minoritized communities. Naming our expectations for contextualized pedagogy around health in adult ELL education should raise important ideological and ethical questions about the role and responsibility many adult ELL teachers take on as decipherers of our healthcare system. For Adkins et al. (1999), teachers should be regarded as "a critical link in a well functioning team of providers" (p. 2), but this coordinated opportunity is relatively rare (…) ESL providers often struggle for their voices to be heard, even as they assume the mandate to assist [learners] in finding their own voices through the medium of English" (p. 2). Public health researchers Rima Rudd and Barbara Moeykens (2002) also express concerns about the capacity of adult education practitioners to address health topics in their teaching. Based on a practitioner survey in the early 2000s, the researchers found that respondents "were cautious about the appropriateness of asking adult education teachers to teach health content. This is not, after all, their area of expertise" (p. 5). Three decades later, these observations remain relevant to efforts to sync adult educational curricula with the "messy, real world of complex care" (Braithwaite, 2018, p. 1).

Even teachers experienced with contextualized instruction may have difficulty anticipating whether and how learners will put new skills to use in the real world. Consider the case of Jing Mei,[3] an English learner and an elder who has lived much of her adult life in a Cantonese-only speaking neighborhood in San Francisco: how can contextualized pedagogy build on the competence that Jing Mei has already honed through interactions with local health services, largely in Cantonese, and identify healthcare tasks where learning English would be useful while supporting her emerging bilingual identity? The idea that Jing Mei will need to learn how to do healthcare tasks in English that she already does in other languages is a flawed assumption. For many linguistically minoritized adults, the ability to navigate health care in the U.S. is a bilingual competence, and contextualized instruction cannot ignore this reality.

Jing Mei's example also illustrates that it is more productive (albeit more challenging) to interpret "context" in terms of how learners *actually* experience the healthcare system in their everyday lives, and not based on an idealized characterization of how the system is meant to be experienced. Seeing the healthcare system through the eyes of our learners is skilled, time-intensive work that goes to the heart of the adult educator's pedagogical expertise (cf., Jacobson et al., 2003). In Jing-Mei's case, her English tutor used an initial needs assessment and learner-generated texts about cooking, favorite foods, using public transportation, and finding information on the Internet to explore her health-related interests and goals for using English.

Teachers' *own* understanding of the healthcare system is also important to consider in implementing contextualized pedagogy around health. In a survey of adult ELL teachers' readiness to integrate the topic of diabetes prevention into their teaching (Santos et al., 2014), teachers were generally enthusiastic but less sure about their ability to track down preventive tools and resources that would be relevant to their learners. The teachers reported wanting more curricular tools and teacher training on diabetes prevention content. While most teachers cited ease with addressing topics such as nutrition, exercise, and the role of social support in diabetes prevention, they were less comfortable addressing "diabetes screenings" or "disease risk factors." This finding signals the need for greater clarity around the extent to which adult ELL teachers should be prepared to interpret risk factors and screening guidelines.

Contextualized pedagogy around health care can bring up feelings of uneasiness or helplessness in teachers if learners share personal experiences of trauma or illness that are painful or shocking to hear (Singleton, 2002). Nash et al. (1992) acknowledge that a teacher will need to "be a careful and responsive listener, picking up on issues that should be further explored, and letting go of the ones that won't be of interest to everyone or that may be too emotionally painful to pursue" (p. 2). Nash et al.'s words are significant for today's teachers, whose own sense of well-being, particularly during this pandemic, undoubtedly affects their capacity as teachers. While there is some research on teachers' own stress and struggles to cope during the COVID-19 pandemic (e.g., Etchells et al., 2021; MacIntyre et al., 2020), teachers' emotional labor in health-contextualized pedagogy warrants greater attention.

Adult ELL programs and improving health literacy levels in the "LEP" population

Concerns about widespread low levels of health literacy in the U.S. have been a notable driver of innovative contextualized pedagogy and teacher training. Before we delve into the concept of health literacy, consider the different connotations of the word "literacy" that are suggested by this short list of quotations and headlines:

1. "90 Million Americans are Burdened with Inadequate Health Literacy" (National Academies of Sciences, Engineering, and Medicine, 2004, April 8)
2. "43 Million American Adults Have 'Low' English Literacy Levels" (Language Magazine, 2019)
3. "We approach literacy as a set of socially organised practices which make use of a symbol system and a technology for producing and disseminating it" (Scribner & Cole, 1981, p. 236).
4. A literacy event is "any occasion in which a piece of writing is integral to the nature of the participants' interactions and their interpretive processes" (Heath, 1982, p. 93).
5. "Literacy is about 'reading the world' not just the 'word'" (Freire & Macedo, 1987, p. 35).

The meaning of "literacy" changes depending on whether we emphasize individual competence (#1, #2), the contexts in which skills are used (#3, #4), or the hope that literacy transforms the way people can participate in the world around them (#5).

This debate about the meaning of literacy is hardly new to educators. Adult educators have been critical of the conflation of "low literacy" with people's intelligence, educational potential, or quality of life; adult literacy scholars emphasize that any evaluation of a learner's skills cannot be separated from the social meanings and values placed on specific language and literacy practices (Purcell-Gates, 2007; Weinstein, 1999; see also Scribner & Cole, 1981). This ideological debate about what "literacies" count and how to measure those changes most relevant to learners themselves is still active in the adult literacy field (Perry et al., 2018; Purcell-Gates et al., 2012; Reder, 2015). The reader may find it rather surprising that dialogue between adult literacy and public health has played a relatively minor role in shaping the theorizing, research, and measurement of health literacy in public health. In fact, the preoccupation with measuring "low health literacy levels" means that, in our efforts to conceptualize health literacy, we have spent relatively less time documenting the strategies (e.g., seeking out help from others), sources of resilience, and problem-solving skills used by individuals with low print literacy or beginning English skills (Cuban & Stromquist, 2009; Pettitt & Tarone, 2006; Purcell-Gates, 2007; Wall, 2017).

In a widely cited 2004 report, *Health Literacy: A Prescription to End Confusion*, **health literacy (HL)** is defined as "the degree to which individuals have the capacity to obtain, process, and understand basic health information and services needed to make appropriate health decisions" (Ratzan & Parker, 2000). This popular definition frames health literacy as a functional or purpose-driven capacity. For example, we read healthcare brochures, prescription labels, or insurance policies using different reading strategies than we would if reading a poem or a work email because our ultimate purpose for reading, writing, and speaking is to make informed healthcare decisions.

For the past couple of decades, a great deal of research and federal funding has been invested in understanding the impact of low functional HL levels. The empirical findings paint a distressing picture of adults who do not read or write in English well, frequently referred to as the "limited English proficient" (LEP) population in this literature. Adults who demonstrate low functional HL are particularly vulnerable to poor outcomes if they are also from "LEP" backgrounds, although there also appear to be some differences within linguistic/ethnic groups (Berkman et al., 2011; Doyle et al., 2017; Sentell & Braun, 2012). Studies on "LEP" populations reveal a sobering array of health disparities, with Becerra et al. (2015) naming "LEP" status as a "significant determinant" of low functional HL. Studies link low HL and "LEP" status with disparities in chronic disease management, greater frequency of medication non-adherence and dosing errors, higher hospitalization rates, poor healthcare access, under-utilization of services, and higher rates of poor self-reported health (Harris et al., 2017; Lee et al., 2021; Masland et al., 2011; Sarkar et al., 2016; Yeheskel & Rawal, 2019). The bleak narrative about U.S. HL levels has also been shaped by several large-scale surveys – the 1992 National Adult Literacy Survey (NALS), the 2003 National Assessment of Adult Literacy (NAAL), and the Program for the International Assessment of Adult Competencies (PIAAC) administered in the U.S. in 2012, 2014, and 2017. These surveys provided further evidence of "alarming rates of low literacy in the United States [and demonstrated] that the population with low health literacy simply did not have the health literacy skills to navigate an ever-changing health care system" (Hohn et al., 2019, p. S2).

Getting beyond functional health literacy

Nutbeam (2000) sought to improve the conceptualization of HL by distinguishing three domains that reflect a progression in skill and competence:

> These different 'types' of literacy characterise the practical application of literacy skills ranging from those needed to be able to function effectively in everyday situations (*functional*), to more advanced cognitive and literacy skills which can be used to actively participate in everyday activities and to apply new information to changing circumstances (*interactive*), through to the most advanced cognitive skills which can be applied to critically analyse information, and to use this information to exert greater control over life events and situations (*critical literacy*).
>
> (p. 2015, emphasis added)

Despite Nutbeam's emphasis on the multi-dimensionality of HL, research and interventions have tended to focus on *functional* outcomes, with less emphasis on *interactive* and *critical* HL outcomes (Chen et al., 2015; Fernández-Gutiérrez et al., 2018; Nutbeam, 2008, 2009). This imbalance reflects a reliance on functional HL tools and comparatively less investment in the development of new interactive/critical HL measurements (Pleasant, 2014).

Perry et al. (2018) interrogate the ideological assumptions about "low-skilled" adults undergirding the emphasis on functionality, asking, "What might be reified or legitimated by describing literacy as *functional*, and what might that modifier ignore or dismiss? (...) Who benefits from viewing adult literacy in terms of functionality, and who might be disadvantaged by this perspective?" (p. 90). Exploring answers to these questions is needed to broaden our understanding of health literacy competence in linguistically minoritized communities. For example, functional HL studies tend not to differentiate between (1) learners who cannot speak English well and (2) learners who cannot speak English well and also do not read/write well enough to complete a written functional HL assessment (Kutner et al., 2007; Santos, 2021). Functional measures also are not able to account for HL as a bilingual competence (Harsch & Santos, forthcoming), nor the help-seeking strategies that adults deploy to overcome their own skills gaps (Cuban, 2006; Wall, 2017).

In a review of HL curricula, Chen et al. (2015) found that ELL programs do not limit their curricular focus to the functional domains; they adjust HL emphases based on learner needs and partnership goals, which the authors characterize as a possible strength in classroom-based intervention: "Although these theoretical differences spell a lack of consensus among program designers and scholars, they also suggest multiple routes for supporting health literacy development" (p. 108). For example, curricula that address interactive HL focus on improving learners' skills for talking to providers or building a social support system; curricula that address critical HL help learners strengthen their capacity as advocates, for themselves and other community members. As another example, in The ESL Diabetes Prevention Project, Santos et al. (2014) found that adult ELL teachers could readily align their current practice with HL outcomes in all three domains as they designed lessons on diabetes prevention. These findings suggest a broader view on HL is critical to understanding learners' diverse HL needs and goals and staying responsive to their real-world experiences.

The promise and challenges of HL partnerships between health and adult education

With the surge in HL research, programs around the U.S. responded with innovative models and initiatives (see Table 5.1). These projects demonstrate an array of partnership configurations, such as between adult education and local research universities, with **federally qualified health care centers** (FQHCs) (community-based clinics that aim to offer low-cost/free health care services and are partially funded by federal block grants) and private health insurance foundations (see Hohn et al., 2019).

As highlighted in Table 5.1, the integration of HL in adult education programs addresses the learning needs of *learners* as well as the capacity of their *teachers* to implement curricular tools and resources (see Rudd, 2002). The learner-oriented activities include English instruction around health content, project-based curricula, and experiential learning opportunities that introduce learners to services and service-providers. Particularly innovative is the

Table 5.1 Examples of U.S.-based health literacy partnerships

Project Description	*Example Funded Activities*
The Anchorage Health Literacy Collaborative (Johnson et al., 2019). A partnership between Alaska Literacy Program (ALP), University of Alaska Anchorage, Providence Health and Services Alaska, and local community organizations; funded by ALP, Providence Health and Services Alaska, National Library of Medicine, Leonard Doak Memorial Scholarship Fund, ongoing	• Development of a Peer Leader Navigator (PLN) program • Stipends for PLNs • Project meetings to discuss community health needs and plan community health presentations
The ESL Diabetes Prevention Project (Santos, et al., 2014). A partnership between The California Diabetes Program, University of California-San Francisco, San Francisco State University, City College San Francisco teachers; funded by National Institutes of Health, Centers for Disease Control and Prevention, 2008–2012	• State-wide survey of adult ELL teachers about their interest and readiness to integrate Type 2 diabetes prevention content into instruction • Professional development meetings • HL lesson planning and implementation in five classrooms
The Florida Health Literacy Initiative. A partnership between the Florida Literacy Coalition and Florida Literacy, English language, and family literacy programs; funded by the Florida Blue Foundation, 2009 to present	• Professional development • HL grants to adult education programs • Development of instructional materials, project-based learning modules • Network-building and resource-sharing across organizations
Health Literacy in Adult Education Settings (The Health Literacy Project) (Chervin et al., 2012). A New England-based project, involving six adult education partners; funded by a healthcare foundation, 2008	• Teacher stipends to attend professional development trainings (Health Literacy Study Circles+) and teach health literacy lessons • Purchase of instructional materials • Field trips to local clinics, farmer's markets • Healthcare presentations and workshops for learners

The Literacy Assistance Center of New York City. A partnership between 75 adult basic education (ABE) program programs and 35 community health centers; funded by private foundations and NY Department of Education, 2003–2010	• Professional development via Health Literacy Study Circles+ • HL curriculum development • Network-building and resource-sharing across organizations • Program evaluation • Learner tours of health centers
Quincy Asian Resources. A partnership between Boston-area non-profit organizations, English language programs; funded by the Boston Medical Center Health Net Plan, ongoing	• English language programming around health themes • Workshops on doctor-patient relationships and health insurance • HL curriculum development for English language classrooms
The Chicago Citywide Literacy Coalition (CCLC), Empowerment-based Health Literacy Project. A partnership between eight adult education organizations, including scaleLit (formerly CCLC), local FQHCs; funded by The Chicago Community Trust, 2016–2018	• Learner tours of FQHCs • Collaborative curriculum development on diverse health topics (e.g., chronic diseases, mental health, provider communication) • Teacher stipends
Health and English as a Second Language Literacy Program (HELP) (Feuerherm et al., 2021). A partnership between University of Michigan-Flint, ACE Community Health, and the Genesee County Hispanic Latino Collaborative; Fint Fresh; funded by University of Michigan-Flint and the W.K. Kellogg Foundation, 2018–2021	• Classes in health literacy, English language, water crisis interventions • Resource website about community partners, environmental health issues, and water testing services • Distribution of fresh produce boxes to participants

Source: Adapted from Hohn et al. (2019).

Alaska Literacy Program (ALP), which created a Peer Leadership Navigator Program that trained learners to promote access to health information and HL skills in their own communities (Johnson et al., 2019). Teacher-oriented activities include assessing teacher readiness and interests to integrate health content and professional development opportunities such as Health Literacy Study Circles and resource-sharing meetings (Chervin et al., 2012).

The programs featured in Table 5.1 also reflect the way educational administrators and directors have championed HL initiatives. Teresa Wagner (2019), the former Director of Health Literacy at The Literacy Coalition of Central Texas, cites funding as one of the most significant barriers to sustainable HL programming in adult education: "Without legislation or organized efforts [at the state level], health literacy program directors also must be contract negotiators and salespersons in addition to completing the health literacy work" (p. S39). After her program ended due to the lack of funding, Wagner helped legislative staff pass a Texas HL bill (HB 3682). Wagner's experience speaks to the kind of professional training and advocacy skills educators need if they want to take on more leadership roles in health equity work. It is also clear that coordinated HL agendas at the state level, with strong funding commitments, increase the likelihood that adult educators and learners can participate in these initiatives.

Is it "health literacy" or "health literacies"?

Even though there is no clear consensus on the conceptualization of "health literacy," the application of the concept appears to be expanding. The phrase is used to index a broad array of decision-making capacities in health care, such as: *cancer health literacy* (Echeverri et al., 2018; Sørensen et al., 2020; Zanchetta et al., 2018); *digital health/e-health literacy* (Consavage Stanley et al., 2022; Harris et al., 2019; Wang et al., 2021); *genetic/genomic literacy* (Abrams et al., 2015); *health insurance literacy* (Yagi et al., 2022); *mental health literacy* (Na et al., 2016); *risk literacy* (Garcia-Retamero et al., 2019). This array suggests that HL is not a unitary, monolithic competence but a competence situated in a particular domain of healthcare tasks and knowledge. There are, in fact, multiple **health literacies**. If we accept this premise, then we must also agree that it is not so productive to talk in broad terms about an adult learner's HL level. Rather, we must ask: *health literacy in* *what context, in what languages, and for what health communicative purpose?* These questions are relevant to adult learners but also to clinicians who are endeavoring to learn their patients' languages (Pilar Ortega, personal communication, May 19, 2022). To what extent do clinicians perform their own health literacies in their first and subsequently learned languages? Critical dialogue about the situatedness of health literacies should benefit both adult education and medical education and support improved practice in both professions.

Into the classroom

In this final section, we address the use of group activities commonly used in beginning-level classrooms to highlight the importance of *talk* and *interaction* when scaffolding learners' engagement around health themes. These activities provide a window into the everyday opportunities we can create for our learners to ask questions, admit confusion, and gain trust in their comprehension skills. We begin by describing a classroom lesson in which the teacher facilitates group work around a bubble-map-making activity.

The teacher writes and circles "People I talk to about my health on the board." Talking out loud to model her thinking, she draws lines extending from the circle and writes "my boss," "God," "my sister in Canada," "We talk about Covid-19." "We speak English, a little Russian." "I ask questions." "We help each other."

The teacher asks, "Who do ***you*** *talk to about health?" and tells the learners that they can write in English or their first language, or draw pictures. The learners share their bubble maps in pairs and practice asking each other questions, such as:*

Who do you talk to?
Do you talk in English? Do you talk in your first language?
Do you talk on the phone? Do you text?

The learners ask questions in English, and then switch to their native languages to give more detailed responses. They walk around the classroom to look at other bubble maps and find similarities and differences in their responses. After the teacher helps the learners notice patterns in their responses, they summarize:

We talk about health with our families.
Some of us talk to our bosses.

> *We talk about Covid-19.*
> *We talk about safety and stress.*
> *We talk in English, Spanish, Russian, and Khmer.*
> *We talk at a park and on the phone. We use WhatsApp.*
> *We ask questions. We help each other.*

The collaborative writing activity leads to spontaneous conversations (in first languages and English). One learner wants to write "nurse" in her bubble map but is unsure about the spelling; with help from another learner, she writes "nurse" so her map is more complete. Several learners mention that their bosses give them Covid-19 safety information. Other learners talk about using WhatsApp to confer with family members in home countries about getting vaccinated. Over the next few lessons, the teacher uses this learner-generated text to review new vocabulary, practice reading fluency, and reinforce sound-letter relationships and word families (alphabetic print literacy skills).

Group work activities, like this bubble map activity, can foster interaction and stimulate meaningful communicative use of English. The activity allows learners to practice giving and getting the same information (*I talk to—. Who do you talk to?)* multiple times in different configurations (pairs, with the teacher, in the larger group), which can boost fluency with new phrases. The bubble map, as a visual aid, allows learners to share ideas without limiting them to what they can say in English.

To a lay observer, the learners may appear to be struggling to use English given the use of the first language; the learners' repeated queries to their classmates, "who do you talk to?" may even appear to be a tedious rote learning exercise. As language educators, we need to be able to articulate how these everyday interactions are relatively small-scale but not trivial resources in health equity work. Here is one possible analysis: this activity promotes a culture of inquiry (Singleton, 2004; Weinstein, 1999) as learners get to talk about where, how, and from whom they get health information. These exchanges enable the teacher to learn about learners' social support systems and encourage them to explore new information outlets. The teacher acts as a facilitator rather than the source of authoritative answers.

The learners focus on asking/answering questions in English while talking about their health information-seeking habits; this activity provides an opportunity for learners to "balance skills and structures with meaning-making and knowledge creation" (Weinstein, 2004, p. 10). Some beginning-level learners are proficient enough to ask opening questions in English but may need to use first languages to explain in detail their help-seeking processes or check their understanding of a peer's answer. This translanguaging (see Chapter 4) supports meaning-making and reflects real-world problem-solving; as Condelli and Wrigley (2006) emphasize, "the problems of real life do not wait for English to catch up" (p. 18).

A lay observer may also ask, does this activity give learners accurate content knowledge about the healthcare system? How about directing them to reliable websites and patient portals so they avoid getting misinformation from friends and social media? While these are valid questions to ask about health communication and help-seeking behaviors, we do not think they are more important than questions about learning and the transfer of skills and knowledge (James, 2018; Perkins & Salomon, 1996; Roumell, 2019). Questions about learning enable us to appreciate how learners, particularly newcomers to the U.S. healthcare system, go about discovering, assembling, and re-assembling their network of sources as their health information needs change over time. It would be misguided to assume that learners need knowledge about available resources *before* they can begin applying help-seeking behaviors. The reality is that learning to assemble a network and using that network are concurrent, mutually reinforcing processes.

The syndemic perspective (introduced in Chapter 1) challenges us to change how we think about language learners, "from seeing learners as individual language producers to seeing them as members of social and historical collectivities" (Norton, 2006, p. 23). Membership in these "collectivities" – as English learners, Facebook users, refugees, parents, and so forth – may open up or close off opportunities to control one's healthcare decision-making. To claim agency in these collectivities, learners need opportunities to actively participate in the production of knowledge. In the bubble-making activity, learners have a relatively low-stakes opportunity to do this: they can ask questions, introduce new ideas, request clarification, and confirm their comprehension. For adults who are emerging bilinguals, the classroom is likely one of the rare places where active participation around health topics in new languages is made possible. Language acquisition research has well established that understanding is a co-constructed phenomenon (Harris, 2005; Hellerman, 2008; Koike, 2003, 2012; Norton & Toohey, 2001; van Lier, 1996). In practice, co-construction is not guaranteed to be an equitable experience: emerging bilingual learners often are "expected to work to understand the native speaker, rather than the native speaker ensuring that the learner understands" (Norton, 2013, p. 78). From this view, classroom instruction should not narrowly focus on ensuring learners' comprehension of healthcare information but rather on strengthening their capacity to shape healthcare interactions, and to that end, "to shape their own learning, to think critically, and to make decisions outside the classroom that may set new directions for their lives" (Wallerstein & Auerbach, 2004, p. 2). There are everyday opportunities in the adult ELL classrooms where this strengthening work is taking place if we commit to seeing classrooms in this role.

Conclusion

The popular discourse around "low-skilled," "LEP" adult learners often narrowly frames learning as a process aimed at closing a skills gap between "native-speaking" and "non-native-speaking" adults. We hope this chapter signals the need for a serious re-boot in our conversations about learning, language, and health outcomes. We have demonstrated that, with rich, contextualized pedagogy organized around healthcare issues that matter to learners, real growth is possible. The classroom provides a space where learners learn new ways of communicating their healthcare needs, using language to ask questions, call out injustices, assert patient rights, or build solidarity with others around common barriers. Classrooms also allow learners to celebrate everyday, incremental learning gains, share frustrations, discover new motivations for learning, and mobilize for change. The syndemic view reminds us that the adult education system alone cannot be responsible for adult learner empowerment in health care. With stronger partnerships between adult education and health care, we are better able to situate learners' motivations to learn new skills and knowledge as part of a broader pursuit of full participation in our healthcare system.

Questions and activities

1. On a scale of 1–5 (5 is very high), how would you assess your capacity and readiness to create contextualized language pedagogy around healthcare issues in learners' lives? What support and resources do you need to strengthen and sustain your capacity and readiness in this regard?
2. If you are a teacher, what activities would you use to address *functional health literacy, interactive health literacy*, and *critical*

health literacy in your teaching? What ideas do you have for supporting and measuring learner gains in all three areas?

3. Where do you see opportunities to link classroom practice to the call for health equity? Who are the learners, colleagues, and community partners whose stories can be integrated into lesson ideas and activities? Drawing on ideas in this chapter, identify 1–2 action steps you can take. Get feedback on your ideas from colleagues in language education and/or health care.

Notes

1 We use "adult English language learner" (ELL) and "adult English as a Second Language (ESL) learne" interchangeably to refer to learners enrolled in classrooms where English acquisition is the primary pedagogical goal. While it is more accurate to refer to beginning-level learners as *emergent bilingual/multilingual learners*, we use the descriptors "adult ELL/ESL" since they are commonly understood by practitioners, researchers, and policymakers.

2 Contextualized pedagogy is a widely valued practice in many areas of second language/additional language education, across many education levels; in this chapter, we are focused on its implementation with adult English language learners.

3 Pseudonym for an English learner in a service-learning tutoring program Maricel supervised in Spring 2021.

6 Strengthening our capacity for health equity work

By the end of this chapter, you will be able to answer these questions:

1. Why are community-engaged partnerships between universities and communities essential to advancing health equity? What are promising examples and models?
2. What kind of support (e.g., professional training, mentorship, time, and funding) do applied linguists need to build this capacity for coalition-building?
3. Am I ready to be a change agent for health equity, and where do I go from here?

Introduction

One evening in early spring 2022, at a café in downtown Wichita, Kansas, Rachel Showstack (second author) and two of the community leaders on the *Alce su voz* (Spanish for "speak out") advisory board assessed the progress of the partnership they had developed over the previous two years. The discussion began with a reflection on each person's reasons for becoming involved in *Alce su voz* and then turned to the centrality of university partnerships in promoting quality bilingual education programming:

> "These are conversations that *must take place.* They *have* to. If you look at the role of what universities provide, I don't see how anyone could not see the value in having these conversations (…) There's such a high demand [for bilingual speakers]. So you're essentially the solution for [language barriers]. If those

DOI: 10.4324/9781003041184-6

conversations aren't taking place at the university level, I don't know who else can provide that." Officer Paul/Pablo Cruz, Hispanic liaison for the Wichita Police Department, Wichita, KS; Advisory Board Member, *Alce su voz*

"I think Paul brings up a good point with University, but how have we fallen so behind? Why are we waiting till it's the university [to offer language classes], right?" Ana López, District 6 Community Services Representative, Evergreen Resource Center, Wichita, KS; Advisory Board Member, *Alce su voz*

Throughout this book, we have aimed to situate the work of applied linguists in the context of U.S. health disparities, specifically looking at ways that our disciplinary knowledge and tools can be used to expose the roots of linguistic inequities in health care and more optimistically contribute to meaningful change. In this closing chapter, we examine our capacity to be effective partners as we imagine working with diverse stakeholder groups, like Ana, a city employee, and Pablo, a law enforcement officer, featured in our opening quotations, as well as healthcare professionals, educators, translators/interpreters, community organizers, adult learners, and patients. It is relatively rare for applied linguists to receive formal training in community partnerships or coalition-building. Our growth as effective partners has emerged only through intense, hands-on experience working with community members. We have endeavored to hone our partnership skills by seeking guidance from mentors, exchanging information and resources, learning from mistakes, and listening to community feedback. We have also had to discover new ways of balancing the pressures of scholarly productivity with the need to invest significant time and energy in developing trusting relationships with community partners.

As outlined in Chapter 1, the promise of the syndemic perspective lies in changing the ways we think about health, disease, and context. The field of applied linguistics must evolve on multiple levels if we are to sustain our focus on health equity. Understanding the syndemic perspective on health disparities is vital to this evolution. This final chapter clarifies our thinking about steps that we can take to work against "the curse of the piecemeal perspective" (Walzer, 2020, n.p.) in health equity work. Understanding the links between our work as applied linguists and a range of social determinants – affordable housing, public safety, digital connectivity, access to healthy food, and others – is crucial if we are to fully address the factors perpetuating inequities for linguistically minoritized communities.

While there are no straightforward solutions here, there are several steps applied linguists can take to get our own house in order, so we are better prepared to contribute to community-based solutions. We begin by reflecting on our connections to communities, specifically how to conceptualize what community partnership can look like in health disparities work. As an example, we highlight the voices of community stakeholders in Wichita, Kansas, who are collaborating with the local public university to address healthcare barriers in the Latinx community. We also offer some recommendations to help readers reflect on the practical opportunities we have to advance health equity.

Renewing a commitment to community partnership in health disparities work

Community partnership is an established approach for tackling social disparities and empowering minoritized communities in the field of applied linguistics (Auerbach, 2002; Avineri et al., 2018; Bucholtz, 2021; Hohn et al., 2019; Warriner & Miller, 2021). The syndemic framework, introduced in Chapter 1, invites us to reflect on our partnership goals and practices. Recall that the syndemic framework examines how the convergence of structural, social, economic, and environmental factors shapes health outcomes (Singer et al., 2017). We are focused on more than just the co-existence of these factors, but rather on the "big picture view," i.e., the synergistic and reinforcing interactions among factors. The syndemic framework deepens our understanding of the interactions between structural barriers to language access/acceptance and other social stressors (e.g., inadequate housing, poor digital access, or immigration status) that worsen the vulnerability for linguistically minoritized groups. If the syndemic framework compels us to consider how health disparities are associated with the clustering of social and environmental factors in communities, we have an important opportunity to reflect on the way we work *in* and *with* communities.

From a syndemic view, we need to re-think how we define "linguistically minoritized community."[1] It may not seem that unusual to define a community based on geography (e.g., a neighborhood), language dominance (e.g., Cantonese-speaking families), or ethnicity (e.g., Latinos/as). However, from the syndemic view, if we rely on these conventional views on community, we may "[miss] the opportunity to examine interactions and dynamic processes that occur within a community" (Boutin-Foster et al., 2022, p. 10), and as a result, fail to recognize key community leaders or other stakeholders who are central to collaborative problem-solving. Also important are the "social connections [that define a community] and how disruptions in community interactions may contribute to adverse outcomes" (ibid., p. 11).

For example, consider the social connections many adult English learners forge with their English teachers and peers in community-based education programs (Hohn & Rivera, 2019; Nash et al., 1992; Weinstein, 2004). When the pandemic shut down schools, many adult English language learners lost touch with this social connection: learners lost reliable access to trusted information and emotional support at a time when so much of the official public health guidance was available only in English and distributed via digital channels. The isolation was particularly acute for elder learners who did not have alternative information channels, such as a school district or an employer. Fortunately, in some community-based programs, teachers and staff mobilized to set up communication channels (e.g., via WhatsApp) and low-tech pedagogical solutions (e.g., mailing packets to learners' home, tutoring via Facetime), although these solutions still did not reliably work for learners with very low English/literacy skills and/or digital access problems (Handley et al., 2022).

On the one hand, this mobilization seems exceptional; on the other hand, from a syndemic view, this potential for mobilization already exists in community-based education settings (see Chapter 5) and can be harnessed to tackle a cluster of disparities (e.g., language barriers, poor connectivity, isolation, and low trust in public health authorities). Partnerships between adult education, public health, and local community members can work at the nexus of multiple social stressors that impede access to critical health guidelines. Had there already been stronger partnerships between public health and the community-based adult education system, might that have helped to offset these stressors for linguistically minoritized communities during the pandemic?

We must seek transformative changes *across* systems, services, and organizations that will improve synergistic interactions and health outcomes. Change is unlikely without strong partnerships that bring together stakeholders across these sectors.

Pursuing community ownership in partnerships

According to Auerbach (2002), a key component of many successful community partnerships is "participant ownership" which emerges "when community members [feel] that the project [is] theirs, when there [is] a shift from outsider to insider control" (p. 7). Our own "self-reflection on how personal perceptions and attitudes [about these labels and their application] shape community narratives is important to developing [solutions] that empower communities and minimize further marginalization, traumatization, or stigmatization" (Boutin-Foster, 2022, pp. 12–13).

Auerbach (2002) highlights key factors that promote community ownership: "(a) involving community members in planning, (b) ensuring nonhierarchical relations between partners, (c) staffing the project with people from the [communities'] linguistic and cultural backgrounds, and (d) promoting leadership by community members" (p. 7). It is best not to view Auerbach's strategies as a checklist of one-time events but rather as guidelines for how to continually cultivate a culture of community ownership. Ongoing conversations, especially ones that communities themselves lead, provide information on issues important to stakeholders, and at the same time, they foster community agency and a shared sense of purpose. Some stakeholders may mistrust the academy due to previous experiences in which academics have taken information from a community without giving anything back (Bastida et al., 2010). Furthermore, they may not share the researchers' emphasis on measuring and documenting outcomes, as they may have experienced frustration or trauma with these administrative processes in other healthcare, education, and legal contexts. Our use of the term "stakeholder" is intentional here and throughout this volume; we wish to recognize that the work we develop within groups of individuals who have a "stake" (or an interest) in its outcomes. This stakeholder-based structure builds trust but cannot be rushed; as applied linguists, we must be clear with ourselves and all of those with whom we collaborate about our purpose and our intentions. We must plan each phase of engagement carefully and collectively so as not to alienate our stakeholders.

Looking closely at community partnership and ownership in *Alce su voz*

This section focuses on a stakeholder engagement project led by Rachel (second author) that ultimately resulted in the creation of the organization *Alce su voz* and an ongoing agenda of advocacy, community education, workforce development, and policy intervention (Showstack et al., 2021). While the project began with university-led conversations, community stakeholders ultimately drove the partnership development and agenda. Rachel, a faculty member at Wichita State University, identified problems with Kansas's language access policies and practices and reached out to colleagues in the Department of Public Health Sciences about how to support health equity for Spanish speakers. Rachel and Glenn (third author), along with clinical partners and public health colleagues, secured a community engagement grant to improve language access that supported coalition-building among local Latinx community stakeholders in Ohio and Kansas.

Rachel convened a team of Latinx community leaders to help plan and facilitate community stakeholder meetings in Wichita, KS; all of the community leaders came from Spanish-speaking families of Mexican origin who had been affected by language access barriers in Kansas at some point in the past. This commonality contributed to a sense of shared purpose and collective advocacy in the broader group. Over two years, the team participated in a series of meetings to share experiences and identify key action steps and plan community outreach events. In the beginning, the *Alce su voz* meetings provided a platform for members – in their role as patients, family members, interpreters, and healthcare workers – to share personal stories revealing the impact of disparities in language access and acceptance. Personal stories that are linked to a broader sociopolitical context are called testimonios, "a form of expression that comes out of intense repression or struggle…an effort by the disenfranchised to assert themselves as political subjects through others, often outsiders, and in the process to emphasize particular aspects of their collective identity" (Acevedo, 2001, p. 13). The sharing of *testimonios* during *Alce su voz* meetings was often spontaneous and unstructured. Sharing led to more sharing, a process that required a flexible meeting agenda. Frequently, an individual's *testimonio* led to a collective demand for change (see Chapter 3 for more discussion).

Verónica, a Wichita resident, shared a *testimonio* about her exasperating interactions with ED staff that led to a dangerous misdiagnosis of her son's appendicitis (see Chapter 3). As Verónica spoke, the room filled with emotion as listeners uttered expressions of disbelief and shock. Verónica ended her *testimonio* with a clear demand:

> *"Necesito que me ayuden, necesito que llegue más allá esto, porque está pasando mucho, en [el hospital local]… los malos diagnósticos de los pacientes."*
>
> (I need you to help me, I need this to go further, because this is happening a lot at [the local hospital]…patient misdiagnoses.)

Verónica's expression of need ("*Necesito que me ayuden, necesito que llegue más allá esto*") captures her **epistemic authority** – an assertion of one's own legitimacy and credibility (Peled, 2018) – in these community meetings. As a listener, Rachel was deeply moved by the urgency with which Verónica expressed a desire for her story to be heard. Making space for the sharing and collective reflection of these *testimonios* enabled the project to keep the community voice at the center of its work, which in turn fostered a sense of ownership over project directions.

In the early months of the COVID-19 pandemic, the dearth of accessible Spanish-language information about the virus was a major concern raised by many of the stakeholders. In response, the team organized outreach to Spanish-speaking communities to provide personal protective equipment and information about safety protocols, testing, and vaccines. These action steps came from the stakeholders themselves, allowing community members to take up leadership roles and direct the planning process.

At the final funded *Alce su voz* stakeholder meeting, Rachel explained that her university team planned to continue working on the project even after the grant ended. Several community members expressed a similar commitment, as captured in this exchange between Cecilia and Verónica.

CECILIA: *Es muy triste que estas reuniones vayan a terminar así. Yo pienso que no debe haber ningún interés personal sobre las tarjetas [de regalo] o cualquier cosa. Esta información es muy importante, vale mucho más de lo que nosotros recibimos. Entonces, mantengámonos informadas sobre la mesa [redonda]…a mí me interesa mucho como paciente. Es muy importante…No hay que cortar estas reuniones. De verdad, yo apoyo que, si ustedes van a seguir con esto, adelante. Yo estoy de acuerdo y yo aquí estoy presente y apoyo. Ningún interés económico personal tengo. Lo que necesito es información y ayuda.*

VERÓNICA: *Yo también. No es por el interés en que nos den nada. Que esto quede huella,…No que obtengamos algo, sino que dejemos huella para que nos puedan escuchar…A mí me encantan los proyectos comunitarios; yo siempre he estado participando en esto porque me encanta convivir con las personas, que podamos aportar un granito de arena para que nuestras voces se sigan escuchando. Cuenten conmigo, de verdad, en lo que yo pueda hacer de mi parte y podemos dejar esa huellita para que las futuras personas no pasen lo que a lo mejor uno pasó. Yo estoy con ustedes.*

English translation:

CECILIA: It is very sad that these meetings are going to end like this. I think that there shouldn't be any personal interest about the [gift] cards or anything. This information is very important, it is much more valuable than what we get. So let's stay informed about the [round]table...I am really interested as a patient. It is very important...We don't have to stop these meetings. Really, I support that, if you are going to continue with this, go for it. I agree and I am here and I support. I don't have any personal economic interest. What I need is information and help.

VERÓNICA: Me too. It's not because of an interest in you giving us anything. We want this to leave a mark...Not for us to get something, but for us to leave a mark so that they can hear us... I love community projects; I have participated in this because I love to share time with others, so that we can contribute a grain of sand so that our voices continue to be heard. Count me in, seriously, whatever I can do and we can leave our mark so that what happened to some of us doesn't happen to future people. I am with you.

Verónica sees the impact of coming together with others ("*convivir con las personas*") on the community's ability to be heard ("*aportar un granito de arena para que nuestras voces se sigan escuchando*"). Her words "*que dejemos huella para que nos puedan escuchar*" (for us to leave a mark so that they can hear us) capture the power of community voice, a voice that "imposes reception on others" (Bourdieu, 1991). Before ending the meeting, stakeholders identified next steps and affirmed their commitment to collaborating, a positive sign that the community felt ownership over the future of *Alce su voz*.

Recommendations for advancing health equity in applied linguistics

By now, we hope you are convinced that applied linguists are poised to advance health equity. At the same time, we have to consider whether the field of applied linguistics is prepared, materially and psychologically, to engage in this work. It is not yet standard practice for the health field to turn to applied linguistics for their input and expertise when designing interventions in linguistically diverse communities. Many applied linguists carry heavy teaching and service loads in their university positions: finding time and resources to build interdisciplinary, collaborative partnerships with health organizations remains a major challenge. Keeping these reality checks in mind, we would like to offer some recommendations for strengthening our capacity as team players in health equity work.

Recommendation 1: Integrate a focus on health disparities in applied linguistics education and training programs

Applied linguistics courses can be used to meaningfully advance health equity in applied linguistics. The range of possible topics is broad, such as health disparities, health humanities, narrative medicine, health communication, risk messaging, and language ideologies in health care. Our teaching in these areas can be strengthened through interdisciplinary connections and collaborations, including guest lectures, cross-listed courses, and interprofessional events for students and faculty in applied linguistics and health professions. Various U.S. universities already offer courses focusing on language and Latinx health in Spanish-language programs; many anthropology programs offer courses on medical anthropology, with courses on health communication found in communication studies programs. However, applied linguistics courses and programs often focus primarily on language learning, with no curricular connection to language in the health context. As Avineri and Martinez (2021) note, while the field of applied linguistics has shifted toward building partnerships to address language-related inequities, teaching in applied linguistics courses has not caught up with these developments.

Sparking students' curiosity about language and health can occur in multiple areas of the undergraduate curriculum. For example, Rachel teaches an honors course, *Language and Community,* open to all majors, on language and community health. The course assignments include a civic engagement project and a research proposal. One of her students wrote an op-ed about the need for accessible Spanish-language mental health information and services and proposed a community-based participatory research project about perspectives on mental health among different generations of Spanish speakers in the U.S. Courses like this one can spark interest in careers in applied linguistics or healthcare careers that include a focus on language access and health equity.

Pre-professional and graduate programs represent another strategic opportunity, especially if students have the opportunity to carry out original capstone or thesis work. Advanced sociolinguistics seminars are good opportunities to support student exploration of dominant language ideologies, language policies, and communication patterns in health care. As they are introduced to sociolinguistic theories and methodological tools, graduate students can examine the infrastructural underpinnings of linguistic equities and poor health outcomes. For example, in Fall 2020, during the first year of the COVID-19 pandemic, the students in Damián Wilson's sociolinguistics course at the University of New Mexico investigated Albuquerque's landscape of public displays of information and health and safety recommendations related to COVID-19 (Peña-Parr, 2021). Spanish-language messages were observed on highway message boards only until May 2020, but the Spanish-language messaging was discontinued before the pandemic was over. These inconsistencies led them to dig deeper, and they eventually uncovered use of artificial intelligence (AI) to translate vaccination websites for the Department of Health. The AI did not have the ability to identify place names in a text and leave them untranslated. While this flaw did not cause problems for names already in Spanish, such as Bernalillo County, it changed English-named counties, rendering "Muelle" from Quay, "Remolino" from Eddy, and "Conceder" from Grant. Wilson and his students engaged in advocacy for the continued dissemination of COVID-19 information in Spanish, resulting in media attention from television and print outlets, and meetings with state and federal politicians. While the freeway signs have not returned to showing Spanish messaging of any kind, the vaccination site was updated as a result of their efforts.

Curricular initiatives are most rewarding when they are tied to local community needs and productively harness the faculty's expertise and students' readiness to learn. Faculty efforts to advance health equity should be valued by their departments and align with university goals regarding social justice. Administrators can make a difference in this work by incentivizing curricular innovation through faculty stipends, release time, and recognition (e.g., support letters in tenure portfolios).

Recommendation 2: Integrate community service learning into applied linguistics programs

Community Service Learning (CSL), "a form of experiential education where learning occurs through a cycle of action and reflection" (Bandy, 2011, n.p), is another promising strategy for integrating a focus on health equity. CSL can take multiple forms, including direct service-learning (e.g., tutoring and health education), indirect service-learning (e.g., brochure translation), research-based service-learning (e.g., helping a clinic conduct a needs assessment), and advocacy-based service-learning (e.g., legislative testimony) (Showstack, 2022; Seifer & Connors, 2007). CSL experiences can provide students with an opportunity to engage with communities directly affected by disparities and to reflect on the real-world clustering of social factors that contribute to these disparities (Charity Hudley et al., 2008; Fitzgerald, 2009; Wurr & Hellebrandt, 2007). At San Francisco State University, Maricel worked with colleagues across departments to integrate CSL into a graduate certificate program in Immigrant Literacies and Community-Based Partnerships. In the program's pilot year, students worked in cross-disciplinary teams to design community-based projects; for example, a team of students from TESOL and nursing designed a training program that brought nurses and language educators together to explore language and power in their professional practice. Students in both disciplines credited the experience for broadening their perspective on health literacy as "a political force and right" (Santos & Landry, 2008, p. 21).

As highlighted in Chapter 3, the use of CSL in the training of new interpreters/translators is another promising application (Showstack, 2021). Through this service-work, advanced bilingual students can reflect on a range of issues related to language access, such as the language patterns that aid communication (e.g., how pain translates across languages), the reliance on volunteer interpreters in health care, local enforcement of Title VI guidelines, and the patience and time involved in co-constructing meaning in clinical interactions.

CSL models, particularly evident in the context of translation/interpretation, involve important legal and ethical considerations. Instructors and community partners may need to check student work to ensure accurate translations, or clinicians may need extra support understanding protocols for working with volunteer interpreters (Showstack, 2021). Legal protections must be in place to protect the university in the (hopefully rare) event that translation/interpreting errors lead to miscommunication about a patient's condition, misdiagnosis, or other injurious outcomes. Health organizations may be reluctant to participate in a partnership if the volunteer interpreter pool shifts from semester to semester. These considerations are daunting but not insurmountable and require a clear articulation of goals and responsibilities between the university and the community site.

CSL models can also be used to promote public awareness of the bi/multilingual experience in our healthcare system. As part of a digital illness narrative project at the University of Texas-Pan American (Martínez & Martin, 2018), students in a Medical Spanish for Heritage Speakers Program documented community members' narratives of illness and disparities, an experience that prompted the students to critically examine their own histories and healthcare privileges. Martínez and Schwartz (2012) also highlight the benefits of service-learning for heritage language speakers volunteering in a health clinic at the U.S.-Mexico border. Students used their bilingual skills to help translate nutrition educational materials and interpret during diabetes education classes. Students gained important insight into the intermingling of standard and non-standard varieties of Spanish in clinical interactions, a translanguaging practice that aided patient comprehension of health directives. Students deepened their respect for local varieties of Spanish and expanded their thinking about bilingual repertoires in health care.

Successful CSL programs require thoughtful planning and institutional support. Practitioners new to service-learning will need professional development on how to build a sustainable CSL program. Even experienced practitioners will need time and resources (e.g., work stipends, release time) to develop CSL courses and reflection activities, and ideally apply for grants to support partnership-building and evaluate impact.[2] A strong team of collaborators – faculty, staff, administrators, students, and community partners – is essential. Most importantly, taking the time to build relationships (especially with community leaders) and understand community healthcare needs, sources of resilience, and linguistic assets should form the foundation of any CSL program.

Recommendation 3: Build a health disparities research agenda in applied linguistics

In recent years, applied linguists have signaled the need for expanding health disparities research in our discipline (Harvey & Koteyko,

2013; Jones, 2013; Martínez, 2020; Martínez et al., 2021; Showstack et al., 2019; Zarcadoolas et al., 2006), but a coordinated research agenda has yet to emerge.[3] We need an agenda to guide collaborations and inform funding priorities at multiple levels. At the federal level, the National Institutes of Health and the Centers for Disease Control and Prevention, major funders of health disparities research, could use the agenda to encourage innovative research on language as a social determinant and the syndemic mechanisms through which language interacts with other social determinants (e.g., social isolation, migration histories, digital connectivity) to influence health outcomes.

Harsch and Santos (forthcoming) argue that a research agenda could motivate a much-needed "multilingual turn" (May 2013) in health disparities work and help to re-position multilinguality as a resource in our healthcare system, not a risk factor (Ortega et al., 2022; cf., Ortega, 2019). We have yet to shed monolingual, English-dominant biases in U.S. health literacy research that tend to presume learning English confers better health outcomes. A coordinated agenda will stimulate debate as to why comparisons to English-only speaking monolinguals (e.g., "native English-speaking patients") tend to be viewed as the benchmark of methodological rigor. This agenda can chart new research into health literacy competence and meaningful interventions in bilingual communities. We envision the development of new measures that capture how language acceptance (see Chapter 1) and multicompetence, i.e., a concept that recognizes multilingual meaning-making and actively rejects the "native-speaker" fallacy (Cook, 2007), are critical resources in the disruption of linguistic inequities in health care. An agenda will provide guidance to early-career applied linguists, including those in doctoral programs, as they set up dissertations on language and health care. The support of flagship organizations, such as the American Association for Applied Linguistics, will ensure that an agenda is developed with input from a broad swath of practitioners. No doubt many community listening sessions will be critical to developing this agenda so that the voices of the community, the multilingual users of our healthcare system, actively shape the kinds of research questions we pursue.

The value of any health disparities research agenda will require critical interrogation of our research dissemination practices. Applied linguists working in academia typically share empirical knowledge via scholarly publications and conference presentations. However, if we expect our findings to reach diverse audiences, not just other applied linguists, we will need to broaden our communication channels and formats (Showstack, forthcoming). If we expect community members to view our findings as accessible, credible, and relevant, we need to be better informed about community expectations for how research is shared (Manzo, 2020). In what languages should research be shared? To what extent is research jargon confusing or useful? In what modalities can findings be disseminated effectively? How do we support community ownership over data interpretation and dissemination processes? Cashman et al. (2008) describe how visual tools (e.g., maps and graphs) provide community partners and researchers with "a common 'language'" that supports collaborative interpretation of findings (p. 1414); these visual tools also enable community partners to lead research presentations to other community members. D'Ignazio (2017) warns that, if we do not actively adopt inclusive dissemination practices, minoritized communities are "far more likely to be discriminated against…or surveilled with data than they are to use data for their own civic ends" (p. 7). The Learners as Data Interpreters initiative (Handley et al., 2009; Santos et al., 2011) is an example of a community-based effort to empower adult learners with tools for critically questioning the stories told with data and discovering the power of their own personal stories as legitimate data sources.

If syndemic-informed research can reveal the need for community-level solutions to health disparities, making our findings relevant and accessible *to* community members is imperative. We must consider a broad array of public-facing genres (e.g., blogs, op-eds, art, data visualizations, social media, legislative testimony, podcasts, videos) for sharing our work (cf. Showstack, forthcoming). We encourage readers to consider which genres best suit your communication strengths and partnership purposes, and then, as needed, hone new dissemination practices. As Krashen (2012) has remarked, "Getting information [about language] to the public and eventually to opinion leaders is a task we must all take part in" (p. 232).

Recommendation 4: Build the field's (and your own) capacity for community partnership

Applied linguists need to develop communication and interpersonal practices that support their authenticity and effectiveness as community partners. As described by Auerbach (2000), "the extent to which [you] are willing to let go of control and genuinely share decision-making with community participants often determines the viability of the partnership" (p. 6). For community projects to thrive, we need to examine the sources of authority that control what it means to be healthy and how "health problems" or "language problems" are defined (Zarcadoolas et al., 2006). The pandemic has undoubtedly taught us that we cannot minimize the importance of trusted biomedical/public health experts, but we must work to ensure that community members are viewed as experts of their healthcare needs and decision-makers in their own right. As community partners, we need to be able to navigate shifts in power in a community engagement project and demonstrate an ability to "welcome unpredictability and diversity" in program goals and implementation (Schofield, 2002, p. 166). Allowing multiple voices to be heard can reveal unexpected priorities and unanticipated action steps. Schofield argues this kind of "wild power" (p. 1590) brings about meaningful change. We saw an example of this "wild power" in the *Alce su voz* project: the public sharing of *testimonios* allowed the community to shape planning discussions and expanded Rachel's understanding of access issues in the community.

How do we grow our capacity to listen empathetically and learn from community voices, particularly when these areas of professional growth are not routinely integrated into most applied linguistics training programs? Throughout the book, we have drawn attention to professional development activities and formats that can support this capacity-building, such as:

- readings on community partnership (e.g., Auerbach, 2002; Avineri et al., 2018; Bucholtz, 2021; Hohn et al., 2019; Warriner & Miller, 2021)
- university coursework that addresses language, health, and health disparities
- service-learning opportunities
- practitioner-led inquiry groups, such as study circles
- community listening sessions on language access
- networking events across community sectors
- professional conferences/webinars in and outside your discipline
- collaborative curriculum planning to design health literacy programs

The catalyst for pursuing professional development may come from your own healthcare experiences, the witnessing of linguistic discrimination in health care, or perhaps the pandemic has exposed access disparities in your communities that cannot be ignored. No matter the point of entry, we hope readers discover meaningful opportunities "to listen and observe, ask questions rather than offer answers, and seek root causes rather than quick fixes" (Safir & Dugan, 2021, p. 61).

Strong leadership in universities, healthcare organizations, local government, and community-based organizations is critically needed. From a syndemic perspective, we need leaders (e.g., directors, deans, managers, legislators, etc.) to champion health equity and to educate themselves about the synergistic interactions that threaten equitable access in linguistically minoritized communities. Ideally, you work for an organization that invests in your growth as a community partner, whether through training, funding (e.g., a conference stipend), or mentorship, but we also recognize that many of us work in institutions and programs where these kinds of material supports are the exception, not the norm.

Recommendation 5: Take steps to boost our grant-writing capacity as applied linguists

Funding is critical if applied linguists wish to be active contributors to health disparities work. Grant-seeking and writing requires coordinated administrative and technical skills, and applied linguists, depending on where they work, may not experience the same level of support as scholars in other fields. For applied linguists who carry heavy teaching and administrative loads, the capacity to write and manage grants is often strained. Applied linguists may not be as familiar with multiple funding streams, such as through the National Institutes of Health, or with panel-based peer-review processes (Bonetta, 2008). Learning to write grant proposals, which is different from writing academic publications (Porter, 2017), can be challenging without professional training and support with the drafting process.

As noted in other recommendations, applied linguists need to be vocal about their professional development needs as grant-writers. Some universities already offer training and resources through offices of sponsored research or faculty development centers, but those resources may be designed for biomedical scientists or public health researchers, and not readily accessible to language professionals. University administrators should proactively survey applied linguistics faculty about their grant-writing needs, orient them to diverse funding streams, and support their grantsmanship. Another critical part of this capacity-building are mentorship programs for applied linguists from historically under-represented backgrounds. This kind of infrastructural investment can begin to address persistent racial disparities in scholarly recognition and funding success in applied linguistics (Bhattacharya et al., 2020) and health (Taffe & Gilpin, 2021).

Recommendation 6: Lift up bilingualism in our healthcare system

Bilingual education scholars Else Hamayan and Rebecca Freeman Field (2012) pose a weighty question to K-12 educational leaders, "What is bilingualism worth, and how much should we be willing to invest in it?" (p. 243). Our final recommendation invites readers to see Field and Hamayan's question in a new light: "What is bilingualism worth *in our U.S. healthcare system*, and how much should we be willing to invest in it?" As Hamayan and Field observe, the fact that we *need* to justify the value of bilingualism reveals how entrenched a monolingual English bias remains in U.S. society, including in our healthcare system. In a study of health and public safety professions, Alarcón et al. (2014) found that "fluent bilinguals receive lower average wages than monolingual English speakers, despite their added linguistic asset" (p. 156). Although investment in interpretation services can reduce healthcare costs in the long run (e.g., Brandl et al., 2020), the loose enforcement of language access policies seems to undervalue bilingualism as a hallmark of quality health care (see Chapter 2). Bilingual physician Pilar Ortega (2022) summarizes the sobering state of affairs:

> The U.S. societal push toward monolingualism has stunted the linguistic growth of our professionals. Despite immigrant families' reliance on their own children's bilingualism to navigate healthcare, the experience of language-based discrimination has caused many to discourage younger generations from pursuing or openly displaying non-English skills....[A] hierarchical perspective has resulted in English functionally dominating academic discourse...Even when medical language programs

> are offered, courses are often student-run without professional guidance or assessment, something that would never be allowed to happen in English clinical education. This linguistic double standard sends the message that for non-English health communication, *un poquito* is good enough.
>
> (p. 1552)

Ortega outlines several action steps in medical schools that are ripe for the collaborative energies of applied linguists: integrate language education into medical training; assess clinicians' language skills prior to any patient interactions; promote academic publishing in languages other than English; and integrate non-dominant varieties into professional linguistic standards. To Ortega's list, we add steps that we can take *within* applied linguistics to elevate bilingualism as a healthcare asset: provide scholarships to bilingual students pursuing careers in language and health; encourage bilingual students to participate in service-learning opportunities in health care; organize mentorship programs that pair early-career bilingual applied linguists with bilingual health disparities researchers[4]; provide career counseling and shadow opportunities for bilingual professionals; publicly recognize the accomplishments of bilingual applied linguists working in health care in popular media. Clearly, no single tactic will bring about an ideological sea-change, but each step helps to clarify the vision of what is needed to uplift bilingualism in health care.

Final reflections

We are only beginning to unpack the range of syndemic-informed applications and intervention routes we can help forge as applied linguists. If we use a syndemic sensibility (Martínez, 2020) to interrogate language, power, and health, how does that shape the kinds of interventions and partnerships we build? If we take as a starting point that language proficiency interacts with other socio-political factors to shape healthcare experiences, how would that change the way we characterize the linguistic profiles of minoritized patient populations? If we hold primary the idea that health disparities are tied to local context, how does that change the way we engage people living and working in those communities? These questions merit serious debate and dialogue in our field, and syndemic theory invites us to see the pursuit of answers as a shared responsibility.

We draw on a parable from Toni Morrison's 1993 Nobel Prize lecture that speaks powerfully about individual and shared responsibility toward language:

> 'Once upon a time there was an old woman. Blind but wise.'... One day the woman is visited by some young people [who doubt her wisdom and seek to test her]... They stand before her, and one of them says, 'Old woman, I hold in my hand a bird. Tell me whether it is living or dead.' She does not answer, and the question is repeated. 'Is the bird I am holding living or dead?'
>
> Still she doesn't answer. She is blind and cannot see her visitors, let alone what is in their hands. She does not know their color, gender or homeland. She only knows their motive.
>
> The old woman's silence is so long, the young people have trouble holding their laughter.
>
> Finally she speaks and her voice is soft but stern. 'I don't know', she says. 'I don't know whether the bird you are holding is dead or alive, but what I do know is that it is in your hands. It is in your hands.'
>
> (Morrison, 1993, pp. 9–11)

Morrison's parable draws attention to a critical moment of choice in our response to linguistic injustice and health disparities: we must consider the different inflection points in our professional and personal lives where there is an opportunity to make choices about how we regard language – "as a living thing, over which we can have control (...) as an act with consequences" (ibid., p. 13). For us, the group in Morrison's parable refers to our professional networks and disciplinary homes, and the woman as the seasoned community leader-partner who recognizes that the answer to the question must be individually *and* collectively owned.

We hope we have showcased the many ways that applied linguists are already responding to "bird-in-hand" moments in their everyday practices. We also hope this book has stirred in you, our reader, a sense of possibility about the areas of need that call you to action.

Questions and activities

1 This chapter highlights several narrative methodologies for honoring the healthcare experiences of linguistically marginalized communities (e.g., *testimonios*, illness narratives, digital

stories). Whose stories about linguistic barriers in health care need greater attention? How might these methodologies be used to lift up those voices?

2 Reflect on the *Alce su soz* project and outline a new project that addresses language barriers in your local community. How can the issues be understood from a syndemic perspective, i.e., in synergistic relation to other social, cultural, linguistic, and/or medical factors? Whose perspectives would you tap into? Who are the stakeholders? What institutions could be called upon to share in the problem-solving?

3 Explore your university's catalogue for courses that address language and health issues (language disciplines, health and medical education, anthropology, sociology, etc.). Identify classes that would be most helpful to your particular interests or issues relevant to local healthcare issues. Are there service-learning classes that support your community work? Are there classes in applied linguists and health disciplines that are ripe for cross-disciplinary innovation, such as syllabus sharing or team-teaching? What new courses that focus on language and health disparities could you propose?

Notes

1 We credit Boutin-Foster et al.'s (2022) insightful report about syndemic perspectives and community engagement in the Jackson Heart Study for helping us refine our own thinking about community partnerships.

2 For CSL resources, see San Francisco State University's Institute of Civic and Community Engagement website: https://icce.sfsu.edu/faculty-staff-resources

3 For examples of efforts to build coordinated research agendas, see Douglas Fir Group (2016), MacSwan (2020), National Academies of Sciences, Engineering, and Medicine (2017), and Patient-Centered Outcomes Research Institute (2022).

4 As part of on-going diversity and inclusion efforts, the American Association for Applied Linguistics offers mentoring and early-career awards that could support this health disparities work.

Afterword

Pilar Ortega

A doctor who speaks "*un poquito de español*" decides not to call for an interpreter because the process would take too long.

A researcher includes limited English proficiency as an exclusion criterion in their clinical trial protocol because of the difficulties in translating informed consent documents and hiring bilingual staff.

A nursing student on their way to study for an exam is asked by a supervisor to stay late at the hospital to serve as an interpreter despite being untrained and uncompensated for that role.

A multilingual clinician is chastised as displaying unprofessional behavior for greeting a colleague in a shared non-English language at work.

An educator is asked to teach Spanish to medical students without compensation because it is an extracurricular activity.

A medical school only hires English-speaking standardized patients for students to practice clinical communication skills because it is challenging to identify and train non-English-speaking actors.

These examples demonstrate linguistic discrimination in action in the healthcare space, and it is a daily reality that I witness in my work as an emergency physician, medical educator, and researcher.

According to the Centers for Disease Control and Prevention, health equity means that every person has the opportunity to attain their full health potential (*Health Equity*, 2022). Providing equitable care to individuals with different needs means that some individuals will require a greater amount of resources, such as time, cost, and services, in order to achieve their best health. When we justify giving substandard care to a group of people – in this case, those who prefer a non-English language – by citing time constraints and lack of resources, we are telling them that they are not deserving of the same quality of care as English speakers. Similarly, when we create and sustain health care and educational systems that neither welcome nor incentivize multilingualism, we are sending a message to all members of linguistically diverse communities – including the multilingual health professional workforce – that *they* are not welcome.

Although I cannot claim to be an applied linguist – my professional training is in the field of medicine – I do think of myself as a *linguistically prepared physician.* Growing up in the United States with a Spanish-speaking family, I learned Spanish first and English once I started school. As a child, I was a cultural and linguistic healthcare navigator for the adults in my family. While pursuing my undergraduate studies, I became a volunteer medical interpreter at a local hospital and took advanced Spanish coursework. When I began learning about patient-doctor communication in medical school, I immediately began taking notes both in English (the language of my training) and in Spanish so I could prepare to provide quality care to the community I wanted to serve. Those notes became the basis for a course I designed and taught to my medical student peers, and, eventually, for my first book – *Spanish and the Medical Interview: A Textbook for Clinically Relevant Medical Spanish.*

Now a board-certified emergency physician, the core of my educational and research work is on patient-centered communication with linguistically diverse populations, with a focus on U.S. Spanish speakers. As one of few Latinas in academic medicine (only 6% of U.S. practicing physicians identify as Hispanic/Latinx [Felida et al., 2021], and even fewer are in academics), I have gladly taken on the responsibility of creating space for language in academic medical discourse. As my work has evolved to include curricular, pedagogical, and assessment components, so has my need (and desire) to expand my knowledge of linguistics as applied to health and healthcare communication.

Nothing has been so instrumental in my own path toward becoming a *linguistically prepared physician* as my interdisciplinary collaborations with applied linguists. Our complementary perspectives have been the source of enriching debate, eye-opening learning experiences, and academic productivity: in the past two years, I have published ten peer-reviewed articles co-authored with applied linguists, and I lead multiple ongoing research studies together with investigators who have linguistic training. In fact, it is precisely to strengthen the connection between professionals with a clinical background and those with linguistic training that I founded a non-profit organization called the National Association for Medical Spanish (NAMS) in 2020. Approximately half of NAMS' professional membership base consists of clinicians and half of language professionals, creating a setting in which interdisciplinary collaboration is the norm.

Through these shared spaces, I have learned that although linguists and clinicians experience very different professional training, the core motivation that leads us to pursue language for medical purposes is almost always the same – to improve health equity. *Health Disparities and the Applied Linguist* brings health equity to the forefront of applied linguistics. Specifically, the book addresses three essential considerations about language in health to which I can personally attest from my work in the field.

First, language in health is more than just an exchange of information. The book broadens our understanding of both what is meant by "language" and what is meant by "health." In so doing, it becomes evident that in order to achieve health equity, we must go beyond language for the purpose of information-gathering and look to language as a means to achieve a bond between clinician and patient and to promote *acceptance*. Educational initiatives that focus on language for exchanging information only may not do justice to how much we can achieve through language. Similarly, attempts to improve care for linguistically diverse patients may fall short if health systems only seek to provide interpreter services and fail to address language-concordant care by qualified bilingual clinicians. Research must look at outcomes beyond access to care and information accuracy and should explore concepts of identity and trust. Moving forward, we must not only focus on interpreters as purely an information conduit but also explore what skills and knowledge are needed for clinicians to provide high-quality language-concordant care and for clinicians and interpreters to collaborate as a healthcare team.

Second, language in health is messy, and that's okay. Language necessarily intersects with other social determinants of health, such as race/ethnicity, immigration status, and economic conditions, among others. The book further challenges the traditional model that suggests that social determinants – including language – have a causative relationship with health outcomes. Instead of a linear oversimplification, we are exposed to the idea of a *syndemic sensibility*, one in which we are asked to consider a less linear and, therefore, more complex interaction between multiple factors, diseases, or health conditions. From a research perspective, this focus on dynamic interaction may be harder to study than the static linear model, but for anyone who has seen language differences play out in the clinical space, it most certainly rings true.

Despite a natural trepidation that may come with the prospect of delving into the messy work of researching language and health as *syndemic*, our fears should be substantially abated by the **third and most important learning point of the book: we are not alone. Language study should not occur in isolation, and neither should medicine.** None of us – whether linguists or clinicians – should take the next steps in the study and advancement of language in health alone. As linguists and clinicians, we need each other, but most importantly, *we need patients and communities.* Patient-centered care is a path toward health equity, not because it is easy, but because it is *real.* It forces us to understand that it is the patient's story, in their words and from their perspective, that matters the most to their accurate diagnosis, appropriate treatment, and best recovery.

In sum, the book teaches us – irrespective of whether our prior training is medical or linguistic – to conceptualize and, therefore, verbalize the connection between language and health equity. For the many linguists and clinicians involved in medical language education who grew up witnessing linguistic injustice in health care, nothing could be more obvious than the connection between language and health. Yet, in order to secure the resources (e.g., funding, institutional support) needed for medical language efforts to be effective and sustainable, we must be able to convincingly explain it to people in positions of power – most of whom do not share our personal lived experiences of injustice.

This book is a toolbox that allows the reader first to understand, through sound arguments and evidence, the inextricable link between language and health. Remember those optical illusion drawings in which some people at first see only one image and do not realize there is a second image as well? (See figure on p. 116.)

Once someone points out the image you missed, you can no longer "unsee" it. It is not, in fact, the revered stethoscope but rather the human connection that connects clinicians and patients as partners in achieving best health. Similarly, once you see the connection that Drs. Santos, Showstack, Martínez, Magaña, and Mr. Colcher have so clearly drawn between language and health equity, you cannot unsee it, and, what's more, you will be eager to share it with others.

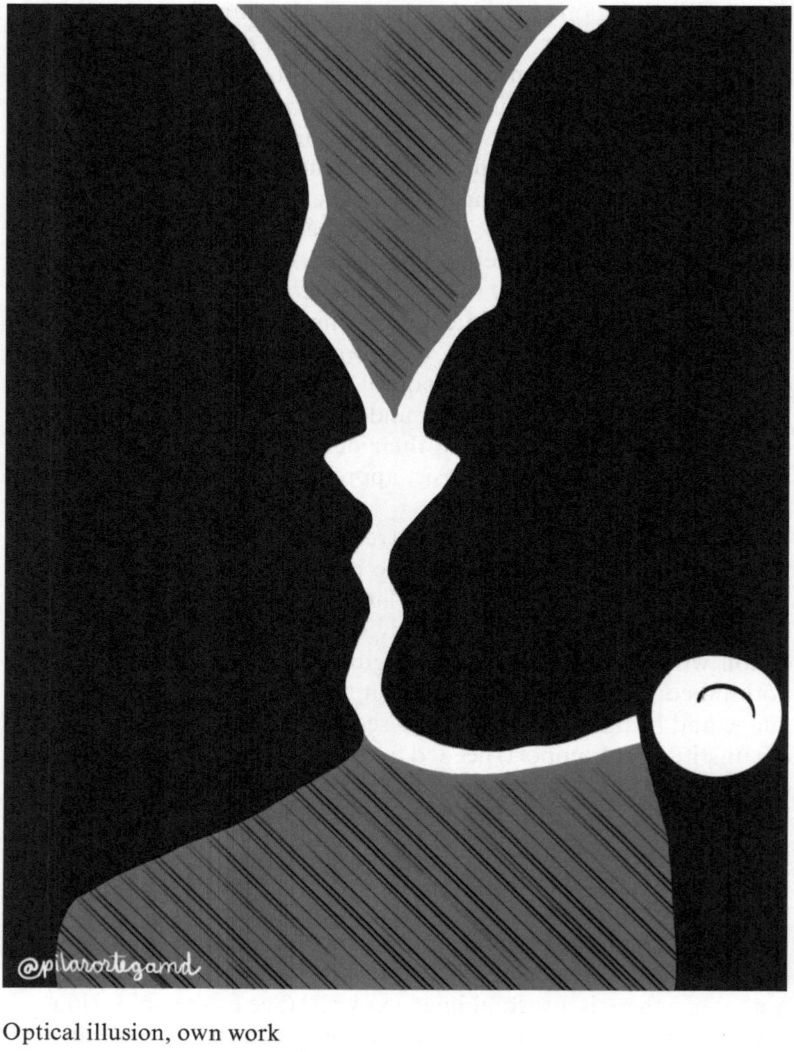

Optical illusion, own work

References

Abraído-Lanza, A. F. (2015). Latino health: A snapshot of key issues. *Health Education & Behavior, 42*(5), 565–568. https://doi.org/10.1177/1090198115606906

Abrams, L. R., McBride, C. M., Hooker, G. W., Cappella, J. N., & Koehly, L. M. (2015). The many facets of genetic literacy: Assessing the scalability of multiple measures for broad use in survey research. *PLoS One, 10*(10). https://doi.org/10.1371/journal.pone.0141532

Acevedo, L. del A. (2001). *Telling to live: Latina feminist testimonios*. Durham: Duke University Press.

Adkins, M., Birman, A., & Sample, B. (1999). *Cultural adjustment: The refugee experience, the role of the teacher, and ESL activities*. Denver, CO: Spring Institute for International Studies.

Ainsworth-Vaughn, N. (1998). *Claiming power in doctor–patient talk*. New York: Oxford University Press.

Alarcón, A., Di Paolo, A., Heyman, J., & Morales, M. C. (2014). Returns to Spanish-English bilingualism in the new information economy: The health and criminal justice sectors in the Texas border and Dallas-Tarrant counties. In R. M. Callahan & P. C. Gándara (Eds.), *The bilingual advantage, language, literacy, and the U.S. labor market* (pp. 138–159). Bristol: Multilingual Matters.

Allison, A., & Hardin, K. (2019). Missed opportunities to build rapport: A pragmalinguistic analysis of interpreted medical conversations with Spanish-speaking patients. *Health Communication, 35*(4), 494–501. https://doi.org/10.1080/10410236.2019.1567446

Altman, M. R., Oseguera, T., McLemore, M. R., Kantrowitz-Gordon, I., Franck, L. S., & Lyndon, A. (2019). Information and power: Women of color's experiences interacting with health care providers in pregnancy and birth. *Social Science & Medicine, 238*(1). https://doi.org/10.1016/j.socscimed.2019.112491

Anzaldúa, G. (1999). *Borderlands/La Frontera* (2nd ed.). San Francisco, CA: Aunt Lute Books.

Arocha, I., & Joyce, L. (2013). Patient safety, professionalization, and reimbursement as primary drivers for national medical interpreter certification in the United States. *The International Journal for Translation and Interpreting Research, 5*(1), 127–142. https://doi.org/10.3316/informit.282664730001770

Auerbach, E. (1992). *Making meaning, making change: Participatory curriculum development or adult ESL literacy.* Washington, DC: Center for Applied Linguistics.

Auerbach, E. (2002). *Community partnerships.* Alexandria, VA: TESOL, Inc.

Avineri, N., & Martinez, D. C. (2021). Applied linguists cultivating relationships for justice: An aspirational call to action. *Applied Linguistics, 42*(6), 1043–1054.

Avineri, N., Graham, L. R., Johnson, E. J., Conley Riner, R., & Rosa, J. D. (Eds.). (2018). *Language and social justice in practice.* New York: Routledge.

Bancroft, M., Garcia-Beyaert, S., Allen, K., Carriera-Contreras, G., & Socarras-Estrada, D. (2016). *The medical interpreter: A foundation textbook for medical interpreting.* Columbia, MD: Language and Culture Press.

Bandy, J. (2011). *What is service learning or community engagement?* Vanderbilt University Center for Teaching. https://cft.vanderbilt.edu/guides-sub-pages/teaching-through-community-engagement/.

Barad, K. (2007). *Meeting the universe halfway: Quantum physics and the entanglement of matter and meaning.* Durham: Duke University Press. https://doi.org/10.1111/j.1527-2001.2009.00013_10.x

Bastida, E. M., Tseng, T.-S., McKeever, C., & Jack, L. (2010). Ethics and community-based participatory research: Perspectives from the field. *Health Promotion Practice, 11*(1), 16–20. https://doi.org/10.1177/1524839909352841

Becerra, M. B., Becerra, B. J., Daus, G. P., & Martin, L. R. (2015). Determinants of low health literacy among Asian-American and Pacific Islanders in California. *Journal of Racial and Ethnic Health Disparities, 2*(2), 267–273. https://doi.org/10.1007/s40615-015-0092-0

Berkman, N. D., Sheridan, S. L., Donahue, K. E., Halpern, D. J., & Crotty, K. (2011). Low health literacy and health outcomes: An updated systematic review. *Annals of Internal Medicine, 155*(2), 97–107. https://doi.org/10.7326/0003-4819-155-2-201107190-00005

Betancourt, H., Flynn, P. M., & Ormseth, S. R. (2011). Healthcare mistreatment and continuity of cancer screening among Latino and Anglo-American women in southern California. *Women & Health, 51*(1), 1–24. https://doi.org/10.1080/03630242.2011.541853

Bhattacharya, U., Jiang, L., & Canagarajah, S. (2020). Race, representation, and diversity in the American Association for Applied Linguistics. *Applied Linguistics, 41*(6), 999–1004. https://doi.org/10.1093/applin/amz003

Bigelow, M., & Vinogradov, P. (2011). Teaching adult second language learners who are emergent readers. *Annual Review of Applied Linguistics, 31*, 120–136. https://doi.org/10.1017/S0267190511000109

Bloom-Pojar, R. (2018). *Translanguaging outside the academy: Negotiating rhetoric and healthcare in the Spanish Caribbean.* Chicago, IL: National Council of Teachers of English.

Bonetta, L. (2008). Enhancing NIH grant peer review: A broader perspective. *Cell, 135*(2), 201–204. https://doi.org/10.1016/j.cell.2008.09.051

Bourdieu, P. (1990). *The logic of practice* (R. Nice, trans.). Stanford, CA: Stanford University Press.

Bourdieu, P. (1991). *Language and symbolic power* (G. Raymond & M. Adamson, trans.). Cambridge, MA: Harvard University Press.

Bourne, J. (2014). "A stone of hope": The Civil Rights Act of 1964 and its impact on the economic status of black Americans. *Louisiana Law Review, 74*(4), 1195–1226.

Boutin-Foster, C., Hastings, J., German, J.R., Hites, L., Eng, E., Turner, E., ... Sutton, V. (2022). Reconsidering community-engaged research through a syndemic theoretical framework: Lessons from COVID-19. *Progress in Community Health Partnerships: Research, Education, and Action, 16*(2), 83–90. doi:10.1353/cpr.2022.0042.

Braithwaite, J. (2018). Changing how we think about healthcare improvement. *BMJ, 361.* https://doi.org/10.1136/bmj.k2014

Brandl, E. J., Schreiter, S., & Schouler-Ocak, M. (2020). Are trained medical interpreters worth the cost? A review of the current literature on cost and cost-effectiveness. *Journal of Immigrant and Minority Health, 22*(1), 175–181. https://doi-org.jpllnet.sfsu.edu/10.1007/s10903-019-00915-4

Braveman, P., & Gottlieb, L. (2014). The social determinants of health: It's time to consider the causes of the causes. *Public Health Reports, 129*(Suppl. 2), 19–31. https://doi.org/10.1177/00333549141291S206.

Brice Heath, S. (1983). *Ways with Words: Language, life and work in communities and classrooms.* Cambridge: Cambridge University Press.

Briggs, C. L. (2019). Language, justice, and rabies: Notes from a fatal crossroads. In N. Avineri, L. Graham, E. Johnson, R. Conley Riner & J. Rosa (Eds.), *Language and social justice in practice* (pp. 109–118). New York: Routledge.

Briggs, C. L., & Mantini-Briggs, C. (2016). *Tell me why my children died: Rabies, indigenous knowledge, and communicative justice.* Durham: Duke University Press.

Brooks, K., Stifani, B., Ramírez Battle, H., Aguilera Nunez, M., Erlich, M., & Diaz, J. (2016). Patient perspectives on the need for and barriers to professional medical interpretation. *Rhode Island Medical Journal, 99*(1), 30–33.

Bucholtz, M. (2021). Community-centered collaboration in applied linguistics. *Applied Linguistics, 42*(6), 1153–1161. https://doi.org/10.1093/applin/amab064

Canagarajah, S. (2013). *Translingual practice: Global Englishes and cosmopolitan relations.* Abingdon: Routledge.

Carter, P. (2014). National narratives, institutional ideologies, and local talk: The discursive production of Spanish in a "new" US Latino community. *Language in Society, 43*(2), 209–240. https://doi.org/10.1017/S0047404514000049

Cashman, S. B., Adeky, S., Allen III, A. J., Corburn, J., Israel, B. A., Montaño, J., Rafelito, A., Rhodes, S. D., Swanston, S., Wallerstein, N., & Eng, E. (2008). The power and the promise: Working with communities to analyze data, interpret findings, and get to outcomes. *American Journal of Public Health, 98*(8), 1407–1417. https://doi.org/10.2105/AJPH.2007.113571

Centers for Disease Control and Prevention, National Center for Chronic Disease Prevention and Health Promotion. (2022, March 3). *Health equity.* https://cdc.gov/chronicdisease/healthequity/index.htm

Cestari, T., Stockler-Rex, S., Runge, D., Remer, C., Meder, D., & Allen, K. (in press). *The remote interpreter.* Columbia, MD: Culture & Language Press.

Chang, H., Hutchinson, C., & Gullick, J. (2019). Pulled away: The experience of bilingual nurses as ad hoc interpreters in the emergency department. *Ethnicity & Health, 26*(7), 1045–1064. https://doi.org/10.1080/13557858.2019.1613518

Chang, P., & Fortier, J. (1998). Language barriers to health care: An overview. *Journal of Health Care for the Poor and Underserved, 1998*(9), S5–S20. https://doi.org/10.1353/hpu.2010.0706

Chao, M., Handley, M., Quan, J., Sarkar, U., Ratanawongsa, N., & Schillinger, D. (2015). Disclosure of complementary health approaches among low income and racially diverse safety net patients with diabetes. *Patient Education and Counseling, 98*(1), 1360–1366. https://doi.org/10.1016/j.pec.2015.06.011

Charity Hudley, A., Harris, J., Hayes, J., Ikeler, K., & Squires, A. (2008). Service-learning as an introduction to sociolinguistics and linguistic equality. *American Speech, 83*(2), 237–251. https://doi.org/10.1215/00031283-2008-016

Chen, A., Youdelman, M., & Brooks, J. (2007). The legal framework for language access in healthcare settings: Title VI and beyond. *Journal of General Internal Medicine, 22*(Suppl. 2), 362–367. https://doi.org/10.1007/s11606-007-0366-2

Chen, J., Fang, H., & Rizzo, J. A. (2011). Physician-patient language concordance and malpractice concerns. *Medical Care, 49*(11), 1040–1044. https://doi.org/10.1097/MLR.0b013e31822efc98

Chen, X., Goodson, P., & Acosta, S. (2015). Blending health literacy with an English as a Second Language curriculum: A systematic literature review. *Journal of Health Communication, 20*(Suppl. 2), 101–111. https://doi.org/10.1080/10810730.2015.1066467

Cheng, E. M., Chen, A., & Cunningham, W. (2007). Primary language and receipt of recommended health care among Hispanics in the United States. *Journal of General Internal Medicine, 22*(Suppl. 2), 283–288. https://doi.org/10.1007/s11606-007-0346-6

Cheng, H. L., Lopez, A., Rislin, J. L., Kim, H. Y., Turner, J., Terhorst-Miller, H., Lopez-Harder, J., & Cha, C. H. (2018). Latino/Hispanic community adults' healthcare experience in a New Mexico borderland region. *Journal of Health Disparities Research and Practice, 11*(4), 68–90. https://digitalscholarship.unlv.edu/jhdrp/vol11/iss4/5

Cherny, N. (2012). Controversies in oncologist-patient communication: A nuanced approach to autonomy, culture, and paternalism. *Oncology, 26*(1), 37–43.

Chervin, C., Clift, J., Woods, L., Krause, E., & Lee, K. (2012). Health literacy in adult education: A natural partnership for health equity. *Health Promotion Practice, 13*(6), 738–746. https://doi.org/10.1177/1524839912437367

Condelli, L., & Wrigley, H. S. (2006). Instruction, language, and literacy: What works study for adult ESL literacy students. *Proceedings from the inaugural LESLLA symposium, Tilburg, Netherlands, August 2005.* https://bit.ly/LESLLA1

Consavage Stanley, K., Harrigan, P. B., Serrano, E. L., & Kraak, V. I. (2022). A systematic scoping review of the literacy literature to develop a digital food and nutrition literacy model for low-income adults to make healthy choices in the online food retail ecosystem to reduce obesity risk. *Obesity Reviews, 23*(4). https://doi.org/10.1111/obr.13414

Cook, V. J. (2007). Multi-competence: Black-hole or worm-hole for second language acquisition research. In Z. Han (ed.), *Understanding second language process* (pp. 16–26). Clevedon: Multilingual Matters.

Cordella, M. (2004). *The dynamic consultation: A discourse analytical study of doctor-patient communication.* Amsterdam: John Benjamins.

Cromley, J. (2000). *Learning to think, learning to learn: What the science of thinking and learning has to offer adult education.* Washington, DC: National Institute for Literacy.

Crossman, K., Wiener, E., Roosevelt, G., Bajaj, L., & Hampers, L. (2010). Interpreters: Telephonic, in-person interpretation and bilingual providers. *Pediatrics, 125*(3), e631–e638. https://doi.org/10.1542/peds.2009-0769

Cuban, S. (2006). Following the physician's recommendations faithfully and accurately: Functional health literacy, compliance, and the knowledge-based economy. *Journal for Critical Education Policy Studies, 4*(2), 220–243.

Cuban, S., & Stromquist, N. P. (2009). "It is difficult to be a woman with a dream of an education": Challenging U.S. adult basic education policies to support women immigrants' self-determination. *Journal for Critical Education Policy Studies,* 7(2). http://jceps.com/?pageID=article&articleID=165

Cuevas, A. G., Dawson, B. A., & Williams, D. R. (2016). Race and skin color in Latino health: An analytic review. *American Journal of Public Health, 106*(12), 2131–2136. https://doi.org/10.2105/AJPH.2016.303452

D'Ignazio, C. (2017). Creative data literacy: Bridging the gap between the data-haves and data-have nots. *Information Design Journal, 23*, 6–18.

Davidson, B. (2014). Diagnosing illness across languages: The role of interpreters in medical discourse. *Proceedings of the Twenty-Third*

Annual Meeting of the Berkeley Linguistics Society: General Session and Parasession on Pragmatics and Grammatical Structure (1997), 23, 62–71. https://doi.org/10.3765/bls.v23i1.1261

Dawes, D. (2020). *The political determinants of health*. Baltimore, MD: Johns Hopkins University Press.

De la Torre, A., & Estrada, A. L. (2015). *Mexican Americans & health: Sana! Sana!* (2nd ed.). Tucson, AZ: University of Arizona Press.

de Saussure, F. (2013). *Course in general linguistics* (R. Harris, trans.). New York: Bloomsbury Academic.

DeCola, A. (2011). Making language access to healthcare meaningful: The need for a federal healthcare interpreters' statute. *Journal of Law and Health, 24*(1), 151–182.

Deeb-Sossa, N. (Ed.). (2019). *Community-based participatory research: Testimonios from Chicana/o studies*. Tucson, AZ: University of Arizona Press.

Desai, P. P., Rivera, A. T., & Backes, E. M. (2016). Latino caregiver coping with children's chronic health conditions: An integrative literature review. *Journal of Pediatric Health Care, 30*(2), 108–120. https://doi.org/10.1016/j.pedhc.2015.06.001

Detz, A., Mangione, C. M., Nunez de Jaimes, F., Noguera, C., Morales, L. S., Tseng, C. H., & Moreno, G. (2014). Language concordance, interpersonal care, and diabetes self-care in rural Latino patients. *Journal of General Internal Medicine, 29*(12), 1650–1656. https://doi.org/10.1007/s11606-014-3006-7

Diamond, L. C., & Jacobs, E. A. (2010). Let's not contribute to disparities: The best methods for teaching clinicians how to overcome language barriers to health care. *Journal of General Internal Medicine, 25*(Suppl. 2), S189–S193. https://doi.org/10.1007/s11606-009-1201-8

Diamond, L., & Reuland, D. (2009). Describing physician language fluency: Deconstructing medical Spanish. *Journal of the American Medical Association, 301*(1), 426–428. https://doi.org/10.1001/jama.2009.6

Diamond, L., Izquierdo, K., Canfield, D., Matsoukas, K., & Gany, F. (2019). A systematic review of the impact of patient-physician non-English language concordance on quality of care and outcomes. *Journal of General Internal Medicine, 34*(8), 1591–1606. https://doi.org/10.1007/s11606-019-04847-5

Diamond, L., Jacobs, E., & Karliner, L. (2020). Providing equitable care to patients with limited dominant language proficiency amid the COVID-19 pandemic. *Patient Education and Counseling, 103*(8), 1451–1452. https://doi.org/10.1016/j.pec.2020.05.028

Diamond, L., Luft, H., Chung, S., & Jacobs, E. (2012). "Does this doctor speak my language?": Improving the characterization of physician non-English language skills. *Health Services Research, 41*(1, pt. 2), 556–569. https://doi.org/10.1111/j.1475-6773.2011.01338.x

Diamond, L., Schenker, Y., Curry, L., Bradley, E., & Fernandez, A. (2008). Getting by: Underuse of interpreters by resident physicians. *Journal of General Internal Medicine, 24*(2), 256–262. https://doi.org/10.1007/s11606-008-0875-7

Diamond, L., Tuot, D., & Karliner, L. (2012). The use of Spanish language skills by physicians and nurses: Policy implications for teaching and testing. *Journal of General Internal Medicine, 27*, 117–123. https://doi.org/10.1007/s11606-011-1779-5

Douglas Fir Group. (2016). A transdisciplinary framework for SLA in a multilingual world. *Modern Language Journal, 100* (Suppl. 2016), 19–47.

Doyle, G., Gibney, S., Quan, J., Martensen, U., & Schillinger, D. (2017). Health literacy, health care utilization, and direct cost of care among linguistically diverse patients with type 2 diabetes mellitus. *Health Literacy Research and Practice, 1*(3), e116–e126. https://doi.org/10.3928/24748307-20170613-01

Dunlap, J., Jaramillo, J., Koppolu, R., Wright, R., Mendoza, F., & Bruzoni, M. (2015). The effects of language concordant care on patient satisfaction and clinical understanding for Hispanic pediatric surgery patients. *Journal of Pediatric Surgery, 50*(9), 1586–1589. https://doi.org/10.1016/j.jpedsurg.2014.12.020

Echeverri, M., Anderson, D., & Nápoles, A. M. (2018). Assessing cancer health literacy among Spanish-speaking Latinos. *Journal of Cancer Education, 33*(6), 1333–1340. https://doi.org/10.1007/s13187-017-1255-y

Erzinger, S. (1991). Communication between Spanish-speaking patients and their doctors in medical encounters. *Culture, Medicine and Psychiatry, 15*, 91–110.

Etchells, Brannen, L., Donop, J., Bielefeldt, J., Singer, E. A., Moorhead, E., & Walderon, T. (2021). Synchronous teaching and asynchronous trauma: Exploring teacher trauma in the wake of Covid-19. *Social Sciences & Humanities Open, 4*(1). https://doi.org/10.1016/j.ssaho.2021.100197

Felida, N., Chu Zhuang, J., Nouri, Z., Dill, M., & Poll, N. (2021, September). *Diversity among Hispanic/Latinx US Physicians.* Association of American Medical Colleges. https://aamc.org/media/56736/download

Fernandez, A., Schillinger, D., Warton, E. M., Adler, N., Moffet, H. H., Schenker, Y., Salgado, M. V., Ahmed, A., & Karter, A. J. (2011). Language barriers, physician-patient language concordance, and glycemic control among insured Latinos with diabetes: The Diabetes Study of Northern California (DISTANCE). *Journal of General Internal Medicine, 26*(2), 170–176. https://doi.org/10.1007/s11606-010-1507-6

Fernández-Gutiérrez, Bas-Sarmiento, P., Albar-Marín, M., Paloma-Castro, O., & Romero-Sánchez, J. (2018). Health literacy interventions for immigrant populations: A systematic review. *International Nursing Review, 65*(1), 54–64.

Feuerherm, E., Showstack, R., Santos, M. G., Martínez, G., & Jacobson, H. (2021). Language as a social determinant of health: Partnerships for health equity. In D. Warriner & E. Miller (Eds.), *Extending applied linguistics for social impact: Cross-disciplinary collaborations in diverse spaces of public inquiry* (pp. 125–148). London: Bloomsbury Publishing.

Fitzgerald, C. (2009). Language and community: Using service learning to reconfigure the multicultural classroom. *Language and Education, 23*(3), 217–231. https://doi.org/10.1080/09500780802510159

Flores, G., Abreu, M., Barone, C. P., Bachur, R., & Lin, H. (2012). Errors of medical interpretation and their potential clinical consequences: A comparison of professional versus ad hoc versus no interpreters. *Annals of Emergency Medicine, 60*(5), 545–553. https://doi.org/10.1016/j.annemergmed.2012.01.025

Flores, G., Barton Laws, M., Mayo, S., Zuckerman, B., Abreu, M., Medina, L., & Hardt, E. (2003). Errors in medical interpretation and their potential clinical consequences in pediatric encounters. *Pediatrics, 111*(1), 6–14. https://doi.org/10.1542/peds.111.1.6

Frank, A. (2013). *The wounded storyteller: Body, illness, and ethics* (2nd ed.). Chicago: University of Chicago Press.

Freire, P., & Macedo, D. P. (1987). *Literacy: Reading the word & the world.* South Hadley, MA: Bergin & Garvey Publishers.

Fricker, M. (2007). *Epistemic injustice: Power & the ethics of knowing.* Oxford: Oxford University Press.

García, O., & Wei, L. (2014). *Translanguaging: Language, bilingualism and education.* London: Palgrave Pivot.

Garcia-Retamero, R., Sobkow, A., Petrova, D., Garrido, D., & Traczyk, J. (2019). Numeracy and risk literacy: What have we learned so far? *The Spanish Journal of Psychology, 22.* https://doi.org/10.1017/sjp.2019.16

Gerteis, M., Edgman-Levitan, S., Daley, J., & Delbanco, T. (Eds.). (2002). *Through the patient's eyes: Understanding and promoting patient-centered care.* Oxford: Wiley.

Givan, R. (2016). *The challenge to change: Reforming health care on the front line in the United States and the United Kingdom.* Ithaca, NY: ILR Press.

González, H. M., Vega, W. A., & Tarraf, W. (2010). Health care quality perceptions among foreign-born Latinos and the importance of speaking the same language. *Journal of the American Board of Family Medicine, 23*(6), 745–752. https://doi.org/10.3122/jabfm.2010.06.090264

Hamayan, E., & Freeman, R. (2012). *English language learners at school: A guide for administrators* (2nd ed.). Baltimore, MD: Caslon Publishing/Brookes.

Handley, M., Santos, M. G., & Bastias, M. J. (2022). *Working with data in adult English classrooms: Lessons learned about communicative justice during the COVID-19 pandemic* [Unpublished manuscript]. Departments of Epidemiology and Biostatistics, University of California San Francisco.

Handley, M., Santos, M. G., & McClelland, J. (2009). Reports from the field: Engaging learners as interpreters for developing health messages: Designing the *Familias sin plomo* English as a second language curriculum project. *Global Health Promotion, 16*(3), 53–58.

Harris, K. A. (2005). Same activity, different focus. *Focus on Basics: Connecting Research and Practice, 8*(A), 7–10.

Harris, K., Jacobs, G., & Reeder, J. (2019). Health systems and adult basic education: A critical partnership in supporting digital health literacy. *Health Literacy Research and Practice, 3*(3), S33–S36. https://doi.org/10.3928/24748307-20190325-02

Harris, L. M., Dreyer, B. P., Mendelsohn, A. L., Bailey, S. C., Sanders, L. M., Wolf, M. S., Parker, R. M., Patel, D. A., Kim, K., Jimenez, J. J., Jacobson, K., Smith, M., & Yin, H. S. (2017). Liquid medication dosing errors by Hispanic parents: Role of health literacy and English proficiency. *Academic Pediatrics, 17*(4), 403–410. https://doi.org/10.1016/j.acap.2016.10.001

Harsch, S., & Santos, M. G. (in press). Are we overlooking language? An applied linguistics perspective on the role of language as a social determinant of health. In P. Ortega, G. Martínez, M. Lor, & S. Ramírez (Eds.), *The handbook of language in public health and healthcare*. Oxford: Wiley.

Hartley, M., & Repede, E. (2011). Nurse practitioner communication and treatment adherence in hypertensive patients. *The Journal for Nurse Practitioners, 7*(8), 654–659. https://doi.org/10.1016/j.nurpra.2011.04.017

Harvey, K., & Koteyko, N. (2013). *Exploring health communication: Language in action*. New York: Routledge.

Haviland, A. M., Elliott, M. N., Hambarsoomian, K., & Lurie, N. (2011). Immunization disparities by Hispanic ethnicity and language preference. *Archives of Internal Medicine, 171*(2), 158–165. https://doi.org/10.1001/archinternmed.2010.499

Heath, S. B. (1982). Protean shapes in literacy events: Ever-shifting oral and literate traditions. In D. Tannen (Ed.), *Spoken and written language: Exploring orality and literacy* (pp. 91–118). Norwood, NJ: Ablex Publishing.

Hellermann, J. (2008). *Social actions for classroom language learning.* Clevedon: Multilingual Matters.

Heritage, J., & Maynard, D. W. (2011). After 30 years, problems and prospects in the study of doctor–patient interaction. In B. A. Pescosolido, J. K. Martin, J. D. McLeod, & A. Rogers (Eds.), *Handbook of sociology of health, illness, and healing: A blueprint for the 21st century* (pp. 323–342). New York: Springer.

Himmelstein, J., Himmelstein, D. U., Woolhandler, S., Bor, D. H., Gaffney, A., Zallman, L., Dickman, S., & McCormick, D. (2021). Healthcare spending and use among Hispanic adults with and without limited English proficiency, 1999–2018. *Health Affairs, 40*(7), 1126–1134. https://doi.org/10.1377/hlthaff.2020.02510

Hohn, M. D., Lawrence, W., McKinney, J., Rosen, D. J., Santos, M. G., Sheppard, R., Smith, G., & Ziskind, A. (2019). Adult basic education: Community health partnerships and health disparities. *Health Literacy Research and Practice, 3*(3), S1–S7. https://doi.org/10.3928/24748307-20181125-01

Hohn, M. D., & Rivera, L. (2019). The impact and outcomes of integrating health literacy education into adult basic education programs in Boston. *Health Literacy Research and Practice, 3*(Suppl. 3), S25–S32. https://doi.org/10.3928/24748307-20190325-01

Holder, E. (2011). *Memorandum for heads of federal agencies, general counsels, and civil rights heads regarding the federal government's renewed commitment to language access obligations under Executive Order 13166.* Washington, DC: Office of the Attorney General.

Holmes, S. (2013). *Fresh fruit, broken bodies: Migrant farmworkers in the United States.* Berkeley, CA: University of California Press.

Hsieh, E. (2008). "I am not a robot!" Interpreters' views of their roles in health care settings. *Qualitative Health Research, 18*(10), 1367–1383. https://doi.org/10.1177/1049732308323840

Hsieh, E. (2018). Reconceptualizing language discordance: Meanings and experiences of language barriers in the U.S. and Taiwan. *Journal of Immigrant and Minority Health, 20*, 1–4. https://doi.org/10.1007/s10903-017-0556-x

Hulme, P. A., Walker, S. N., Effle, K. J., Jorgensen, L., McGowan, M. G., Nelson, J. D., & Pratt, E. N. (2003). Health-promoting lifestyle behaviors of Spanish-speaking Hispanic adults. *Journal of Transcultural Nursing, 14*(3), 244–254. https://doi.org/10.1177/1043659603014003011

Hunt, D. (2016). *New 2016 ACA rules significantly affect the law of language access* [memo]. Critical Measures e-Learning. https://cmelearning.com/new-2016-aca-rules-significantly-affect-the-law-of-language-access/

Hymes, D. (1997). The scope of sociolinguistics. In N. Coupland & A. Jaworski (Eds.), *Sociolinguistics: A reader and coursebook* (pp. 12–22). New York: Palgrave.

Islam, M. M. (2019). Social determinants of health and related inequalities: Confusion and Implications. *Frontiers in Public Health, 7*(11). https://doi.org/10.3389/fpubh.2019.00011

Jacobs, E. A., Karavolos, K., Rathouz, P. J., Ferris, T. G., & Powell, L. H. (2005). Limited English proficiency and breast and cervical cancer screening in a multiethnic population. *American Journal of Public Health, 95*(8), 1410–1416. https://doi.org/10.2105/AJPH.2004.041418

Jacobson, E., Degener, S., & Purcell-Gates, V. (2003). *Creating authentic materials and activities for the adult literacy classroom: A handbook for practitioners.* Boston, MA: National Center for the Study of Adult Language Learning and Literacy. https://ncsall.net/fileadmin/resources/teach/jacobson.pdf

James, M. (2018). Teaching for transfer of second language learning. *Language Teaching, 51*(3), 330–348. https://doi.org/10.1017/S0261444818000137

Jaramillo, J., Snyder, E., Dunlap, J. L., Wright, R., Mendoza, F., & Bruzoni, M. (2016). The Hispanic Clinic for Pediatric Surgery: A model to improve parent-provider communication for Hispanic pediatric surgery patients. *Journal of Pediatric Surgery, 51*(4), 670–674. https://doi.org/10.1016/j.jpedsurg.2015.08.065

John-Baptiste, A., Naglie, G., Tomlinson, G., Alibhai, S. M., Etchells, E., Cheung, A., Kapral, M., Gold, W. L., Abrams, H., Bacchus, M., & Krahn, M. (2004). The effect of English language proficiency on length of stay and in-hospital mortality. *Journal of General Internal Medicine, 19*(3), 221–228. https://doi.org/10.1111/j.1525-1497.2004.21205.x

Johnson, R. M., Shepard, L., Van Den Berg, R., Ward-Waller, C., Smith, P., & Weiss, B. D. (2019). A novel approach to improve health literacy in immigrant communities. *Health Literacy Research and Practice, 3*(Suppl. 3), S15–S24. https://doi.org/10.3928/24748307-20190408-01

Jones, R. H. (2013). *Health and risk communication: An applied linguistic perspective.* New York: Routledge.

Jost, T. (1994). Medicare and the Joint Commission on accreditation of healthcare organizations: A healthy relationship? *Law and Contemporary Problems, 57*(4), 15–45. https://doi.org/10.2307/1192055

Jost, T. (2020, June 17). *Rule cutting ACA's transgender, other civil rights protections called into question by Supreme Court* [blog post]. California Health Care Foundation. https://chcf.org/blog/rule-cutting-acas-transgender-other-civil-rights-protections-called-into-question-supreme-court/

Juckett, G. (2013). Caring for Latino patients. *American Family Physician, 87*(1), 48–54.

Kam, J. A., & Lazarevic, V. (2014). The stressful (and not so stressful) nature of language brokering: Identifying when brokering functions as a cultural stressor for Latino immigrant children in early adolescence. *Journal of Youth and Adolescence, 43*(12), 1994–2011. https://doi.org/10.1007/s10964-013-0061-z

Kamimura, A., Chernenko, A., Nourian, M., Aguilera, G., Assasnik, N., & Ashby, J. (2016). The role of health literacy in reducing negative perceptions of breast health and treatment among uninsured primary care patients. *Journal of Community Health, 38*, 858–863. https://doi.org/10.1007/s10900-013-9669-x

Keers-Sanchez, A. (2003). Mandatory provision of foreign language interpreters in health care services. *The Journal of Legal Medicine, 24*, 557–578. https://doi.org/10.1080/714044490

Keith, K. (2020a, June 13). *HHS strips gender identity, sex stereotyping, language access protections from ACA anti-discrimination rule* [blog post]. Health Affairs Blog. https://healthaffairs.org/do/10.1377/hblog20200613.671888/full/

Keith, K. (2020b, June 16). *Supreme court finds LGBT people are protected from employment discrimination: Implications for the ACA* [blog post]. Health Affairs Blog. https://healthaffairs.org/do/10.1377/hblog20200615.475537/full/

Kelly, N. (2008). The voice on the other end of the phone. *Health Affairs, 27*(6), 1701–1706. https://doi.org/10.1377/hlthaff.27.6.1701

Khanijou, S. (2005). Rebalancing healthcare inequities: Language service reimbursement may ensure meaningful access to care for LEP patients. *DePaul Journal of Healthcare Law, 9*(1), 855–884.

King-Ramírez, C., & Martínez, G. (2018). Nurses' perspectives on language standardization in health care: The silencing of bilingual health providers. *Heritage Language Journal, 15*(3), 297–318. https://doi.org/10.46538/hlj.15.3.2

Koh, H., Berwick, D., Clancy, C., Baur, C., Brach, C., Harris, L., & Zerhusen, E. (2012). New federal policy initiatives to boost health literacy can help the nation move beyond the cycle of costly "crisis care". *Health Affairs, 31*(2), 434–443. https://doi.org/10.1377/hlthaff.2011.1169

Koike, D. (2003). La construcción del significado en el español: Elementos pragmáticos de la interacción dialógica. In D. Koike (Ed.), *La co-construcción del significado en el español de las Américas: Acercamientos discursivos* (pp. 11–24). Ottawa: Legas.

Koike, D. (2012). Variation in NS-learner interactions: Frames and expectations in pragmatic co-construction. In C. Félix-Brasdefer & D. Koike (Eds.), *Pragmatic variation in first and second language contexts: Methodological issues* (pp. 175–208). Amsterdam: John Benjamins.

Krashen, S. (2012). What are some key elements in advocating for educational programs for English language learners? In E. Hamayan & R. Freeman Field (Eds.), *English language learners at school: A guide for administrators* (2nd ed., pp. 229–232). Philadelphia, PA: Caslon.

Kutner, M., Greenberg, E., Jin, Y., Boyle, B., Hsu, Y., Dunleavy, E., & National Center for Education Statistics. (2007). *Literacy in everyday life: Results from the 2003 National Assessment of Adult Literacy*. NCES 2007–490. National Center for Education Statistics.

Lang, E. V. (2012). A better patient experience through better communication. *Journal of Radiology Nursing, 31*(4), 114–119. https://doi.org/10.1016/j.jradnu.2012.08.001

Language Magazine. (2019, September 10). *43 million American adults have 'low' English literacy levels.* https://languagemagazine.com/2019/09/10/43-million-in-u-s-have-low-literacy-levels/

Lee, E., & Canagarajah, S. (2019). The connection between transcultural dispositions and translingual practices in academic writing. *Journal of Multicultural Discourses, 14*(1), 14–28. https://doi.org/10.1080/17447143.2018.1501375

Lee, M., Lee, M. A., Ahn, H., Ko, J., Yon, E., Lee, J., Kim, M., & Braden, C. J. (2021). Health literacy and access to care in cancer screening among Korean Americans. *Health Literacy Research and Practice, 5*(4), e310–e318. https://doi.org/10.3928/24748307-20211104-01

Leemann Price, E., Pérez-Stable, E. J., Nickleach, D., López, M., & Karliner, L. S. (2012). Interpreter perspectives of in-person, telephonic, and videoconferencing medical interpretation in clinical encounters. *Patient Education and Counseling, 87*(2), 226–232. https://doi.org/10.1016/j.pec.2011.08.006

Leong, M., & Santos, M. G. (2019.) Taking our seat at the table: Why the expertise of LESLLA educators is needed in the health literacy field. *Proceedings from the 9th annual Low Educated Second Language and Literacy Acquisition (LESLLA) Symposium, 2017, Portland, OR* (pp. 53–68). https://bit.ly/LESLLA9

Lindsay, J. (2005). Achieving compliance with Title VI of the Civil Rights Act of 1964: A comprehensive approach to ensuring meaningful access to services for Limited-English-Proficient individuals. *Journal of Nursing Law, 10*(1), 47–55.

López, B. G., Lezama, E., & Heredia, D. (2019). Language brokering experience affects feelings toward bilingualism, language knowledge, use, and practices: A qualitative approach. *Hispanic Journal of Behavioral Sciences, 41*(4), 481–503. https://doi.org/10.1177/0739986319879641

Lozada-Oliva, M. (2017). *Peluda*. Minneapolis, MN: Button Poetry (E-book).

MacIntyre, P. D., Gregersen, T., & Mercer, S. (2020). Language teachers' coping strategies during the Covid-19 conversion to online teaching: Correlations with stress, wellbeing and negative emotions. *System, 94*. https://doi.org/10.1016/j.system.2020.102352

MacSwan, J. (2020). Academic English as standard language ideology: A renewed research agenda for asset-based language education. *Language Teaching Research, 24*(1), 28–36. https://doi.org/10.1177/1362168818777540

Magaña, D. (2019). Cultural competence and metaphor in mental healthcare interactions: A linguistic perspective. *Patient Education and Counseling, 102*(12), 2192–2198. https://doi.org/10.1016/j.pec.2019.06.010

Magaña, D. (2020). Local voices on health care communication issues and insights on Latino cultural constructs. *Hispanic Journal of Behavioral Sciences, 42*(3), 300–323. https://doi.org/10.1177/0739986320927387

Magaña, D. (2021). *Building confianza: Empowering Latinos through transcultural health communication*. Columbus, OH: The Ohio State University Press. https://doi.org/10.26818/9780814214817

Manzo, R. (2020). *Cultura y corazón: A decolonial methodology for community engaged research*. Tucson, AZ: University of Arizona Press.

Margulies, P. (1981). Bilingual education, remedial language instruction, Title VI, and proof of discriminatory purpose: Suggested approach. *Columbia Journal of Law and Social Problems, 17*(1), 99–162.

Marmot, M. (2005). *The status syndrome: How social standing affects our health and longevity.* New York: Henry Holt.

Martínez, G. (2010). Language and power in healthcare: Towards a theory of language barriers among linguistic minorities in the United States. In J. Watzke & P. Chamness Miller (Eds.), *Readings in Language* (Volume 2, pp. 59–74). St. Louis, MO: International Society for Language Studies.

Martínez, G. (2013). Política e ideología del lenguaje en la atención sanitaria para hispanohablantes en los Estados Unidos. In D. Dumitrescu (Ed.), *El español en los Estados Unidos: E pluribus unum?* (pp. 233–250). New York: Academia Norteamericana de la Lengua Española.

Martínez, G. (2020). *Spanish in health care: Policy, practice and pedagogy in Latino health.* New York: Routledge.

Martínez, G., Dejbord-Sawan, P., Magaña, D., Showstack, R., & Hardin, K. (2021). Pursuing testimonial justice: Language access through patient-centered outcomes research with Spanish speakers. *Applied Linguistics, 42*(6), 1110–1124. https://doi.org/10.1093/applin/amab060

Martínez, G., & Martín, K. S. (2018). Language and power in a medical Spanish for heritage learners program: A *Learning by Design* perspective. In G. Zapata & M. Lacorte (Eds.), *Multiliteracies pedagogy and language learning* (pp. 107–128). Camden: Palgrave Macmillan.

Martínez, G., & San Martín, K. (2018). Language and power in a medical Spanish for heritage learners program: A learning by design perspective. In G. C. Zapata & M. Lacorte (Eds.), *Multiliteracies pedagogy and language learning: Teaching Spanish to heritage speakers* (pp. 107–128). New York: Palgrave Macmillan.

Martínez, G., & Schwartz, A. (2012). Elevating "low" language for high stakes: A case of critical, community-based Learning in a Medical Spanish for heritage learners program. *Heritage Language Journal, 9*(2), 37–49.

Martínez, G., Showstack, R., Magaña, D., Hardin, K., Dejbord-Sawan, P., San-Martin, K., & Santos, M. (2020, May 20). *Reclaiming language access in U.S. Latino communities during COVID-19: Patient-centeredness at risk?* [Webinar presented through Ohio State University]. https://u.osu.edu/languageaccessresearch/

Masland, M., Kang, S., & Ma, Y. (2011). Association between limited English proficiency and understanding prescription labels among five ethnic groups in California. *Ethnicity & Health, 16*(2), 125–144. https://doi.org/10.1080/13557858.2010.543950

May, S. (Ed.). (2013). *The multilingual turn: Implications for SLA, TESOL, and bilingual education*. New York: Taylor & Francis Group.

Mayo, R., Parker, V., Sherrill, W., Coltman, K., Hudson, M., Nichols, C., Yates, A., & Pribonic, A. (2016). Cutting corners: Provider perceptions of interpretation services and factors related to use of an ad hoc interpreter. *Hispanic Health Care International, 14*(2), 73–80. https://doi.org/10.1177/1540415316646097

McClellan, S., Wu, F., & Snowden, L. (2012). The impact of threshold language assistance programming on the accessibility of mental health services for persons with limited English proficiency in the Medi-Cal setting (brief report). *Medical Care, 50*(6), 554–558. https://doi.org/10.1097/MLR.0b013e3182463432

McKinney, J., & Santos, M. G. (2019). Putting the literacy back in health literacy: Interventions in U.S. adult literacy and English language programs. In O. Okan, U. Bauer, P. Pinheiro, D. Zamir-Levin & K. Sørensen (Eds.), *International handbook of health literacy* (pp. 387–400). Bristol: Policy Press, University of Bristol.

Metzger, R. (1993). Hispanics, health care, and Title VI of the Civil Rights Act of 1964. *Kansas Journal of Law & Public Policy, 3*(2), 31–42.

Michael, D. (1995). Federal agency use of audited self-regulation as a regulatory technique. *Administrative Law Review, 47*(2), 171–254.

Moran, R. (2005). Undone by law: The uncertain legacy of *Lau v. Nichols. Berkeley La Raza Law Journal, 16*(1), 1–10.

Moran, R. (2009). The untold story of *Lau v. Nichols*. In M. Lacorte & J. Leeman (Eds.), *Español en Estados Unidos y otros contextos de contacto: Sociolingüística, ideología y pedagogía* (pp. 277–302). Madrid: Iberoamericana/Vervuert.

Morrison, T. (1993). *The Nobel Lecture in Literature, 1993*. New York: Alfred A. Knopf.

Na, S., Ryder, A. G., & Kirmayer, L. J. (2016). Toward a culturally responsive model of mental health literacy: Facilitating help-seeking among East Asian immigrants to North America. *American Journal of Community Psychology, 58*(1–2), 211–225. https://doi.org/10.1002/ajcp.12085

Naeem, S. B., & Bhatti, R. (2020). The Covid-19 'infodemic': A new front for information professionals. *Health Information and Libraries Journal, 37*(3), 233–239. https://doi.org/10.1111/hir.12311

Nápoles, A., Santoyo-Olsson, J., Karliner, L., O'Brien, H., Gregorich, S., & Perez-Stable, E. (2010). Clinician ratings of interpreter mediated visits in underserved primary care settings with ad hoc, in-person professional, and video conferencing modes. *Journal of Health Care for the Poor and Underserved, 21*(1), 301–317. https://doi.org/10.1353/hpu.0.0269

Nash, A., Cason, A., Rhum, M., McGrail, L., & Gomez-Sanford, R. (1992). *Talking shop: A curriculum sourcebook for participatory adult ESL*. McHenry, IL: Delta Systems.

National Academies of Sciences, Engineering, and Medicine. (2004, April 8). *90 million Americans are burdened with inadequate health literacy: IOM report calls for national effort to improve health literacy*. https://nationalacademies.org/news/2004/04/90-million-americans-are-burdened-with-inadequate-health-literacy-iom-report-calls-for-national-effort-to-improve-health-literacy

National Academies of Sciences, Engineering, and Medicine. (2017). *Communicating science effectively: A research agenda*. Washington, DC: The National Academies Press. doi: 10.17226/23674.

Ngo-Metzger, Q., Sorkin, D. H., Phillips, R. S., Greenfield, S., Massagli, M. P., Clarridge, B., & Kaplan, S. H. (2007). Providing high-quality care for limited English proficient patients: The importance of language concordance and interpreter use. *Journal of General Internal Medicine, 22*(Suppl. 2), 324–330. https://doi.org/10.1007/s11606-007-0340-z

Nguyen, P. V., Naleppa, M., & Lopéz, Y. (2021). Cultural competence and cultural humility: A complete practice. *Journal of Ethnic & Cultural Diversity in Social Work, 30*(3), 273–281.

Norton, B. (2013). *Identity and language learning: Extending the conversation*. Bristol: Multilingual Matters.

Norton, B., & Toohey, K. (2001). Changing perspectives on good language learners. *TESOL Quarterly, 35*(2), 307–322. https://doi.org/10.2307/3587650

Nutbeam, D. (2000). Health literacy as a public health goal: A challenge for contemporary health education and communication strategies into the 21st century. *Health Promotion International, 15*(3), 259–267. https://doi.org/10.1093/heapro/15.3.259

Nutbeam, D. (2008). The evolving concept of health literacy. *Social Science & Medicine, 67*(12), 2072–2078. https://doi.org/10.1016/j.socscimed.2008.09.050

Nutbeam, D. (2009). Defining and measuring health literacy: What can we learn from literacy studies? *International Journal of Public Health, 54*(5), 303–305. https://doi.org/10.1007/s00038-009-0050-x

Oberlander, J. (2010). Long time coming: Why health reform finally passed. *Health Affairs, 29*(6), 1112–1116. https://doi.org/10.1377/hlthaff.2010.0447

Ortega, L. (2019). SLA and the study of equitable multilingualism. *The Modern Language Journal, 103*, 23–38. https://doi.org/10.1111/modl.12525.

Ortega, P. (2018). Spanish language concordance in U.S. medical care: A multifaceted challenge and call to action. *Academic Medicine, 93*(9), 1276–1280. https://doi.org/10.1097/ACM.0000000000002307

Ortega, P. (2022). Letter to the editor in response to "My son, my Interpreter". *Journal of General Internal Medicine, 37*, 1552. https://doi.org/10.1007/s11606-021-07181-x

Ortega, P., Diamond, L., Alemán, M. A., Fatás-Cabeza, J., Magaña, D., Pazo, V., Pérez, N., Girotti, J. A., & Ríos, E. (2020). Medical Spanish standardization in US medical schools: Consensus statement from a multidisciplinary expert panel. *Academic Medicine, 95*(1), 22–31. https://doi.org/10.1097/ACM.0000000000002917

Ortega, P., & Prada, J. (2020). Words matter: Translanguaging in medical communication skills training. *Perspectives on Medical Education, 9*(4), 251–255. https://doi.org/10.1007/s40037-020-00595-z

Ortega, P., Shin, T. M., & Martínez, G. A. (2022). Rethinking the term "Limited English Proficiency" to improve language-appropriate healthcare for all. *Journal of Immigrant and Minority Health, 24*(3), 799–805. https://doi.org/10.1007/s10903-021-01257-w

Otheguy, R., García, O., & Reid, W. (2015). Clarifying translanguaging and deconstructing named languages: A perspective from linguistics. *Applied Linguistics Review, 6*(3), 281–307. https://doi.org/10.1515/applirev-2015-0014

Parker, M. M., Fernández, A., Moffet, H. H., Grant, R. W., Torreblanca, A., & Karter, A. J. (2017). Association of patient-physician language concordance and glycemic control for limited-English proficiency Latinos with type 2 diabetes. *JAMA Internal Medicine, 177*(3), 380–387. https://doi.org/10.1001/jamainternmed.2016.8648

Parrish, B. (2019). *Teaching adult English language learners: A practical introduction* (2nd ed.). Cambridge: Cambridge University Press.

Patient-Centered Outcomes Research Institute. (2022, March 8). *PCORI proposed research agenda.* https://pcori.org/sites/default/files/PCORI-Proposed-Research-Agenda-English.pdf

Peled, Y. (2018). Language barriers and epistemic injustice in healthcare settings. *Bioethics, 32*, 360–367.

Peña-Parr, V. (2021, November 3). *Life-or-death: An assessment of COVID-19 messaging in New Mexico and potential consequences for the Spanish-speaking population* [paper presentation]. Shared Knowledge 2018 conference, University of New Mexico, Albuquerque, NM.

Peña, P., Stockler-Rex, S., & Cestari, T. (2019, November 21). *Volume II: Video remote interpretation in hospital language access plans* [blog post]. Cloudbreak Health. https://cloudbreak.us/2019/11/21/vri_in_language_access_plans/

Penaranda, E., Diaz, M., Noriega, O., & Shokar, N. (2012). Evaluation of health literacy among Spanish-speaking primary care patients along the US-Mexico border. *Southern Medical Journal, 105*(7), 334–338. https://doi.org/10.1097/SMJ.0b013e31825b2468

Pennycook, A. (2007). *Global Englishes and transcultural flows.* New York: Routledge. https://doi.org/10.4324/9780203088807

Pennycook, A. (2018). *Posthumanist applied linguistics.* London: Routledge. https://doi.org/10.4324/9781315457574-1

Perkins, D., & Salomon, G. (1996). Learning transfer. In A. Tuijnman (Ed.), *International encyclopedia of adult education and training* (pp. 422–427). Oxford: Pergamon Press.

Perry, K. H., Shaw, D. M., Ivanyuk, L., & Tham, Y. S. S. (2018). The "Ofcourseness" of functional literacy: Ideologies in adult literacy. *Journal of Literacy Research, 50*(1), 74–96. https://doi.org/10.1177/1086296X17753262

Pettitt, N., & Tarone, E. (2015). Following Roba: What happens when a low-educated adult immigrant learns to read. *Writing Systems Research, 7*(1). https://doi.org/10.1080/17586801.2014.987199

Plain Writing Act, 5 U.S.C. §1–7 (2010). https://govinfo.gov/content/pkg/PLAW-111publ274/pdf/PLAW-111publ274.pdf

Pleasant, A. (2014). Advancing health literacy measurement: A pathway to better health and health system performance. *Journal of Health Communication, 19*(12), 1481–1496. https://doi.org/10.1080/10810730.2014.954083

Porter, R. (2017). Reprint 2007: Why academics have a hard time writing good grants proposals. *Journal of Research Administration, 48*(1), 15–25.

Purcell-Gates, V. (Ed.). (2007). *Cultural practices of literacy: Case studies of language, literacy, social practice, and power.* Mahwah, NJ: Lawrence Erlbaum Associates.

Purcell-Gates, V., Anderson, J., Gagne, M., Jang, K., Lenters, K. A., & McTavish, M. (2012). Measuring situated literacy activity. *Journal of Literacy Research*, *44*(4), 396–425. https://doi.org/10.1177/1086296X12457167

Rampton, Ben. (2018). *Crossing: Language and ethnicity among adolescents*. New York: Routledge.

Ratzan, S. C., & Parker, R. M. (2000). Introduction. In C. R. Selden, M. Zorn, S. C. Ratzan & R. M. Parker (Eds.), *National library of medicine current bibliographies in medicine: Health literacy* (pp. 19–30). Bethesda, MD: National Institutes of Health, U.S. Department of Health and Human Services.

Raymond, C. W. (2014a). Conveying information in the interpreter-mediated medical visit: The case of epistemic brokering. *Patient Education and Counseling, 97*(1), 38–46. https://doi.org/10.1016/j.pec.2014.05.020

Raymond, C. W. (2014b). Epistemic brokering in the interpreter-mediated medical visit: Negotiating "patient's side" and "doctor's side" knowledge. *Research on Language and Social Interaction, 47*(4), 426–446. https://doi.org/10.1080/08351813.2015.958281

Reardon, S., & Owens, A. (2014). 50 Years after *Brown*: Trends and consequences of school segregation. *Annual Review of Sociology, 40*(1), 199–218. https://doi.org/10.1146/annurev-soc-071913-043152

Reder, S. (2013). Lifelong and life-wide adult literacy development. *Perspectives on Language and Literacy, 39*(2), 18–21.

Reder, S. (2015). Expanding emergent literacy practices: Busy intersections of context and practice. In M. G. Santos & A. Whiteside (Eds.), *Low educated second language and literacy acquisition: Proceedings of the ninth symposium* (pp. 1–29). San Francisco, CA: Lulu Publishing.

Reid, T. (2010). *The healing of America: A global quest for better, cheaper, and fairer health care*. New York: Penguin.

Rodriguez, J. A., Saadi, A., Schwamm, L. H., Bates, D. W., & Samal, L. (2021). Disparities in telehealth use among California patients with limited English proficiency. *Health Affairs, 40*(3), 487–495. https://doi.org/10.1377/hlthaff.2020.00823

Rosenbaum, S., & Schmucker, S. (2017). Viewing health equity through a legal lens: Title VI of the 1964 Civil Rights Act. *Journal of Health Politics, Policy, and Law, 42*(5), 771–788. https://doi.org/10.1215/03616878-3940423

Roumell, E. A. (2019). Priming adult learners for learning transfer: Beyond content and delivery. *Adult Learning, 30*(1), 15–22. https://doi.org/10.1177/1045159518791281

Rudd, R. (2002). A maturing partnership. *NCSALL Focus on Basics, 5*(C). http://ncsall.net/index.html@id=247.html

Rudd, R., & Moeykens, B. (2002). *Adult educators' perceptions of health issues and topics in adult basic education programs*. Cambridge, MA: The National Center for the Study of Adult Learning and Literacy.

Safir, S., & Dugan, J. (2021). *Street data: A next-generation model for equity, pedagogy, and school transformation*. Thousand Oaks, CA: Corwin.

Salgado-Robles, F., & Lamboy, E. M. (2019). The learning and teaching of Spanish as a heritage language through community service learning in New York City. *Revista Signos. Estudios de Lingüística, 52*(101), 1057–1077.

Sanchez-Birkhead, A. C., Kennedy, H. P., Callister, L. C., & Miyamoto, T. P. (2011). Navigating a new health culture: Experiences of immigrant Hispanic women. *Journal of Immigrant and Minority Health, 13*(6), 1168–1174. https://doi.org/10.1007/s10903-010-9369-x

Santos, M. G. (2021, March 20–23). *Finding "low-literate populations" in U.S. health literacy research: A review of labels, descriptors, and measures* [paper presentation]. American Association for Applied Linguistics, Annual Meeting, Virtual.

Santos, M., & Landry, L. (2008). Partners in training: A cross-disciplinary approach to preparing adult literacy practitioners and health professionals. *Focus on Basics, 9*(B), 21–25.

Santos, M. G., Handley, M. A., Omark, K., & Schillinger, D. (2014). ESL participation as a mechanism for advancing health literacy in immigrant communities. *Journal of Health Communication, 19*(Suppl. 2), 89–105.

Santos, M. G., McClelland, J., & Handley, M. (2011). Language lessons on immigrant identity, food culture, and the search for home. *TESOL Journal, 2*(2), 203–228.

Sarkar, M., Asti, L., Nacion, K., & Chisolm, D. (2016). The role of health literacy in predicting multiple healthcare outcomes among Hispanics in a nationally representative sample: A comparative analysis by English proficiency levels. *Journal of Immigrant & Minority Health, 18*(3), 608–615. https://doi.org/10.1007/s10903-015-0211-3

Schenker, Y., Karter, A. J., Schillinger, D., Warton, E. M., Adler, N. E., Moffet, H. H., Ahmed, A. T., & Fernandez, A. (2010). The impact of limited English proficiency and physician language concordance on reports of clinical interactions among patients with diabetes: The DISTANCE study. *Patient Education and Counseling, 81*(2), 222–228. https://doi.org/10.1016/j.pec.2010.02.005

Schenker, Y., Wang, F., Selig, S. J., Ng, R., & Fernandez, A. (2007). The impact of language barriers on documentation of informed consent at a hospital with on-site interpreter services. *Journal of General Internal Medicine, 22*(Suppl. 2), 294–299. https://doi.org/10.1007/s11606-007-0359-1

Schiaffino, M., Al-Amin, M., & Schumacher, J. (2014). Predictors of language service availability in U.S. hospitals. *International Journal of Health Policy and Management, 3*(5), 259–268.

Schiaffino, M., Nara, A., & Mao, L. (2016). Language services in hospitals vary by ownership and location. *Health Affairs, 35*(8), 1399–1407. https://doi.org/10.15171/ijhpm.2014.95

Schofield, A. (2002). Wild power: School-community partnerships in a South African school district. In E. Auerbach (Ed.), *Community partnerships* (pp. 159–169). Alexandria, VA: TESOL, Inc.

Scribner, S., & Cole, M. (1981). *The psychology of literacy.* Cambridge, MA: Harvard University Press.

Seifer, S. D., & Connors, K. (Eds.). (2007). *Community-campus partnerships for health: Faculty toolkit for service-learning in higher education.* Scotts Valley, CA: National Service Learning Clearinghouse. https://www.vanderbilt.edu/oacs/wp-content/uploads/sites/140/faculty-toolkit-for-service-learning.pdf

Sentell, T., & Braun, K. L. (2012). Low health literacy, limited English proficiency, and health status in Asians, Latinos, and other racial/ethnic groups in California. *Journal of Health Communication, 17*(Suppl. 3), 82–99. https://doi.org/10.1080/10810730.2012.712621

Sentell, T., Shumway, M., & Snowden, L. (2007). Access to mental health treatment by English language proficiency and race/ethnicity. *Journal of General Internal Medicine, 22*(Suppl. 2), 289–293. https://doi.org/10.1007/s11606-007-0345-7

Shin, T., Ortega, P., & Hardin, K. (2021). Educating clinicians to improve telemedicine access for patients with limited English proficiency. *Challenges, 12*(34), 1–7. https://doi.org/10.3390/challe12020034

Showstack, R. (in press). Open science and accessible research. In L. Plonsky (Ed.), *Open science in applied linguistics.* Amsterdam: John Benjamins.

Showstack, R. (2019a). *Past injustices and present experiences in medical Spanish service-learning for Spanish heritage speakers.* In invited colloquium *Medical Spanish for Heritage Learners: From context of instruction to curriculum design* [paper presentation]. 6th National Symposium on Spanish as a Heritage Language (NSSHL), University of Texas, Rio Grande Valley, February 2019.

Showstack, R. (2019b). Patients don't have language barriers; the health care system does. *Emergency Medicine Journal, 36*(10), 580–581. https://doi.org/10.1136/emermed-2019-208929

Showstack, R. (2021). Making sense of the interpreter role in a healthcare service-learning program. *Applied Linguistics, 42*(1), 93–112. https://doi.org/10.1093/applin/amz058

Showstack, R. (2022). Audiovisual assignments as service-learning for social justice in Latinx communities. *Spanish as a Heritage Language, 2*(1) https://doi.org/10.5744/shl.2022.1005

Showstack, R., & Guzman, K. (2020). Heritage speakers, monolingual policies, and Spanish language maintenance in Kansas. In S. Alvord & G. Thompson (Eds.), *Contact, community, and connections: Current approaches to Spanish in the United States and Spanish in contact with other languages* (pp. 187–205). Wilmington, DE: Vernon Press.

Showstack, R., Duque, S., Keene Woods, N., López, A., & Chesser, A. (2021). Lifting the voices of Spanish-speaking Kansans: A community-engaged approach to health equity. *Multilingua, 41*(4), 489–517. https://doi.org/10.1515/multi-2021-0082

Showstack, R., Santos, M., Feuerherm, E., Jacobson, H., & Martínez, G. (2019). *Language as a social determinant of health: An applied linguistics perspective on health equity (AAALetter)*. American Association for Applied Linguistics. https://aaal.org/news/language-as-a-social-determinant-of-health-an-applied-linguistics-perspective-on-health-equity

Singer, M. (2009). *Introduction to syndemics: A critical systems approach to public and community health*. San Francisco, CA: Josey Bass.

Singer, M., Bulled, N., Ostrach, B., & Mendenhall, E. (2017). Syndemics and the biosocial conception of health. *Lancet (London, England), 389*(10072), 941–950. https://doi-org.jpllnet.sfsu.edu/10.1016/S0140-6736(17)30003-X

Singleton, K. (2002). ESOL Teachers: Helpers in Health Care. *Focus on Basics, 5*(C), 26–30. https://www.ncsall.net/index.html@id=242.html

Singleton, K. (2004). *Picture stories for adult ESL health literacy*. Center for Applied Linguistics, The Center for Adult English Language Acquisition. https://www.cal.org/caela/esl_resources/Health/healthindex.html

Slade, D., Scheeres, H., Manidis, M., Iedema, R., Dunston, R., Stein-Parbury, J., Matthiessen, C., Herke, M., & McGregor, J. (2008). Emergency communication: The discursive challenges facing emergency clinicians and patients in hospital emergency departments. *Discourse & Communication, 2*(3), 271–298.

Snowden, L., & McClellan, S. (2013). Spanish-language community-based mental health treatment programs, policy-required language-assistance programming, and mental health treatment access among Spanish-speaking clients. *American Journal of Public Health, 103*(9), 1628–1623. https://doi.org/10.2105/AJPH.2013.301238

Sørensen, K., Makaroff, L. E., Myers, L., Robinson, P., Henning, G. J., Gunther, C. E., & Roediger, A. E. (2020). The call for a strategic framework to improve cancer literacy in Europe. *Archives of Public Health, 78*. https://doi.org/10.1186/s13690-020-00441-y

Soto Mas, F., Cordova, C., Murrietta, A., Jacobson, H., Ronquillo, F., & Helitzer, D. (2015). A multisite community-based health literacy intervention for Spanish speakers. *Journal of Community Health, 40*, 431–438. https://doi.org/10.1007/s10900-014-9953-4

Stableford, S., & Mettger, W. (2007). Plain language: A strategic response to the health literacy challenge. *Journal of Public Health Policy, 28*, 71–93. https://doi.org/10.1057/palgrave.jphp.3200102

Stabler, R. (2013). What we've got here is failure to communicate: The plain writing act of 2010. *Journal of Legislation, 40*(2), 280–323.

Steinberg, E. M., Valenzuela-Araujo, D., Zickafoose, J. S., Keiffer, E., & Decamp, L. R. (2016). The "battle" of managing language barriers in health care. *Clinical Pediatrics, 55*(14), 1318–1327. https://doi.org/10.1177/0009922816629760

Stubbe, D. E. (2020). Practicing cultural competence and cultural humility in the care of diverse patients. *Focus, 18*(1), 49–51. https://doi.org/10.1176/appi.focus.20190041

Sudore, R., Landefield, C., Pérez-Stable, E., Bibbins-Domingo, K., Williams, B., & Schillinger, D. (2009). Unraveling the relationship between literacy, language proficiency, and patient-physician communication. *Patient Education and Counseling, 75*(3), 398–402. https://doi.org/10.1016/j.pec.2009.02.019

Taffe, M. A., & Gilpin, N. W. (2021). Racial inequity in grant funding from the US National Institutes of Health. *eLife, 10*, e65697. https://doi.org/10.7554/eLife.65697

Tang, G., Lanza, O., Rodriguez, F. M., & Chang, A. (2011). The Kaiser Permanente clinician cultural and linguistic assessment initiative: Research and development in patient-provider language concordance. *American Journal of Public Health, 101*(2), 205–208. https://doi.org/10.2105/AJPH.2009.177055

Tervalon, M., & Murray-García, J. (1998). Cultural humility versus cultural competence: A critical distinction in defining physician training outcomes in multicultural education. *Journal of Health Care for the Poor and Underserved, 9*(2), 117–125. https://doi.org/10.1353/hpu.2010.0233

The Joint Commission. (2010). *Advancing effective communication, cultural competence, and patient- and family-centered care: A roadmap for hospitals.* Oakbrook Terrace, IL: The Joint Commission.

Thornbury, S. (2015, March 22). *I is for Intersubjectivity.* From An A-Z of ELT [Blog]. https://scottthornbury.wordpress.com/2015/03/22/i-is-for-intersubjectivity/

Tipton, R., & Furmanek, O. (2016). *Dialogue interpreting: A guide to interpreting in public services and the community.* London: Routledge.

Tran, H., & Bhattarai, D. (2014). From *Lau v. Nichols* to the Affordable Care Act: Forty years of ensuring meaningful access in health care for limited English proficient Asian Americans, Native Hawaiians, and Pacific Islanders. *Asian American Policy Review, 24*(1), 7–23.

Traylor, A. H., Schmittdiel, J. A., Uratsu, C. S., Mangione, C. M., & Subramanian, U. (2010). Adherence to cardiovascular disease medications: Does patient-provider race/ethnicity and language concordance matter? *Journal of General Internal Medicine, 25*(11), 1172–1177. https://doi.org/10.1007/s11606-010-1424-8

U.S. Department of Education Office of Career, Technical, and Adult Education. (2021). *Table 507.20: Participants in state-administered adult basic education, adult secondary education, and English as a second language programs, by type of program and state or jurisdiction, selected fiscal years, 2000 through 2018.* https://nces.ed.gov/programs/digest/d20/tables/dt20_507.20.asp

U.S. Department of Education. (n.d.). *The skills that matter in adult education: Defining the approaches that work.* U.S. Department of Education

Literacy Information and Communication System. https://lincs.ed.gov/sites/default/files/DefineApproachesThatWork-508.pdf
U.S. Department of Health and Human Services Office for Civil Rights. (2000). Title VI of the Civil Rights Act of 1964: Policy guidance on the prohibition against national origin discrimination as it affects persons with Limited English Proficiency. *The Federal Register, 65*(169), 52762–52774.
U.S. Department of Health and Human Services Office of Minority Health. (2013). *National standards for Culturally and Linguistically Appropriate Services in health and health care: A blueprint for advancing and sustaining CLAS policy and practice.* Washington, DC: U.S. Department of Health and Human Services.
U.S. Department of Health and Human Services Office of Minority Health. (2001). *National standards for Culturally and Linguistically Appropriate Services in health care.* Washington, DC: U.S. Department of Health and Human Services.
U.S. Department of Health and Human Services. (2013). *Enforcement success stories involving persons with limited English proficiency: Summary of selected OCR compliance reviews and complaint investigations.* https://hhs.gov/civil-rights/for-providers/compliance-enforcement/examples/limited-english-proficiency/index.html
U.S. Department of Health and Human Services. (2020a). *Section 1557 of the Patient Protection and Affordable Care Act: Fact sheet.* https://hhs.gov/civil-rights/for-individuals/section-1557/index.html
U.S. Department of Health and Human Services. (2020b). Nondiscrimination in health and health education programs or activities, delegation of authority. *The Federal Register, 85*(119), 37160–37248.
U.S. Department of Health and Human Services. (n.d.). *Social determinants of health.* https://health.gov/healthypeople/priority-areas/social-determinants-health
U.S. Department of Justice. (2000). *Enforcement of Title VI of the Civil Rights Act of 1964: National origin discrimination against persons with Limited English Proficiency* [Notice]. https://lep.gov/executive-order-13166
U.S. Department of Justice. (2002). Guidance to federal financial assistance recipients regarding Title VI prohibition against national origin discrimination affecting Limited English Proficient persons. *The Federal Register, 67*(117), 41455–41472.
van Lier, L. (1996). *Interaction in the language curriculum: Awareness, autonomy, and authenticity.* London: Longman.
Wagner, T. (2019). Incorporating health literacy into English as a Second Language classes. *Health Literacy Research and Practice, 3*(3), S37–S41. https://doi.org/10.3928/24748307-20190405-02
Wall, T. (2017). *Literacy and its implications for LESLLA immigrant women in Canada* [unpublished capstone project]. Hamline University, St. Paul, Minnesota.
Wallerstein, N., & Auerbach, E. (2004). *Problem-posing at work: Popular educator's guide.* Edmonton, CA: Grassroots Press.

Walqui, A. (2006). Scaffolding instruction for English Language Learners: A conceptual framework. *International Journal of Bilingual Education and Bilingualism, 9*(2), 159–180. https://doi.org/10.1080/13670050608668639

Walzer, C. (2020). COVID-19 and the curse of piecemeal perspectives. *Frontiers in Veterinary Science, 23.* https://doi.org/10.3389/fvets.2020.582983

Wang, C., Wu, X., & Qi, H. (2021). A comprehensive analysis of e-health literacy research: Focuses and trends. *Healthcare, 10*(1). https://doi.org/10.3390/healthcare10010066

Warriner, D., & Miller, E. (Eds.) (2021). *Extending applied linguistics for social impact: Cross-disciplinary collaborations in diverse spaces of public inquiry.* London: Bloomsbury Publishing.

Watt, K., Abbott, P., & Reath, J. (2016). Developing cultural competence in general practitioners: An integrative review of the literature. *BMC Family Practice, 17.* https://doi.org/10.1186/s12875-016-0560-6

Weinstein, G. (1999). *Learners' lives as curriculum.* McHenry, IL: Delta Systems.

Weinstein, G. (2004). Learner-centered teaching in the age of accountability. *CATESOL Journal, 16*(1), 97–110.

Willen, S. S., Knipper, M., Abadía-Barrero, C. E., & Davidovitch, N. (2017). Syndemic vulnerability and the right to health. *The Lancet, 389,* 964–977. https://doi.org/10.1016/S0140-6736(17)30261-1

Willison, C., & Singer, P. (2017). Repealing the Affordable Care Act essential health benefits: Threats and obstacles [editorial]. *American Journal of Public Health, 107*(8), 1225–1226. https://doi.org/10.2105/AJPH.2017.303888

Wodak, R. (1996). *Disorders of discourse.* London: Longman.

Wood, D., Bruner, J., & Ross, G. (1976). The role of tutoring in problem solving. *Journal of Child Psychology and Psychiatry, 17*(2), 89–100.

World Health Organization. (n.d.). Frequently asked questions. Retrieved from http://www.who.int/suggestions/faq/en/

Wrigley, H. (2008). From survival to thriving: Toward a more articulated system for adult English language learners. In I. van de Craats & J. Kurvers (Eds.), *Low-educated adult second language literacy acquisition: Proceedings of the 4th Symposium, Antwerp, Belgium* (pp. 170–183). Utrecht, The Netherlands: LOT. *https://bit.ly/LESLLA4*

Wrigley, H., & Guth, G. (1992). *Bringing literacy to life: Issues and options in adult ESL literacy.* San Mateo, CA: Aguirre International.

Wurr, A., & Hellebrandt, J. (Eds.). (2007). *Learning the language of global citizenship : Service-learning in applied linguistics.* Bolton, MA: Anker Pub.

Wynia, M., & Osborn, C. (2010). Health literacy and communication quality in health care organizations. *Journal of Health Communication, 15*(Suppl. 2), 102–115. https://doi.org/10.1080/10810730.2010.499981

Yagi, B. F., Luster, J. E., Scherer, A. M., Farron, M. R., Smith, J. E., & Tipirneni, R. (2022). Association of health insurance literacy with health care utilization: A systematic review. *Journal of General Internal Medicine, 37*(2), 375–389. https://doi-org.jpllnet.sfsu.edu/10.1007/s11606-021-06819-0

Yeager, K. A., & Bauer-Wu, S. (2013). Cultural humility: Essential foundation for clinical researchers. *Applied Nursing, 26*(4), 1–12. https://doi.org/10.1016/j.apnr.2013.06.008

Yearby, R. (2014). When is change going to come?: Separate and unequal treatment in health care fifty years after the Title VI of the Civil Rights Act of 1964. *SMU Law Review, 67*(2), 287–340.

Yearby, R. (2015). Sick and tired of being sick and tired: Putting an end to separate and unequal health care in the United States 50 years after the Civil Rights Act of 1964. *Health Matrix: Journal of Law and Medicine, 25*(1), 1–32.

Yeheskel, A., & Rawal, S. (2019). Exploring the 'patient experience' of individuals with limited English proficiency: A scoping review. *Journal of Immigrant and Minority Health, 21*(4), 853–878. http://doi.org/10.1007/s10903-018-0816-4

Youdelman, M. (2008). The medical tongue: U.S. laws and policies on language access. *Health Affairs, 27*(2), 424–433. https://doi.org/10.1377/hlthaff.27.2.424

Zanchetta, M. S., Maheu, C., Gebremariam, A. G., Baribeau, P., Ndiaye, N. L., Tamouro, S., Lemonde, M., & Cloos, P. (2018). Immigrant grandmothers' and mothers-in-law's cancer literacy within their family context. *Journal of Women & Aging, 30*(6), 467–483. https://doi.org/10.1080/08952841.2017.1313028

Zarcadoolas, C., Pleasant, A. F., & Greer, D. S. (2006). *Advancing health literacy: A framework for understanding and action*. San Francisco, CA: Jossey-Bass.

Zhao, Y., Segalowitz, N., Voloshyn, A., Chamoux, E., & Ryder, A. G. (2021). Language barriers to healthcare for linguistic minorities: The case of second language-specific health communication anxiety. *Health Communication, 36*(3), 334–346. https://doi.org/10.1080/10410236.2019.1692488

Index